W9-AOW-333

Diane Irons'

14 Day Beauty BOOT CAMP

The Crash Course for Looking and Feeling Great!

SOURCEBOOKS MEDIAFUSION™
AN IMPRINT OF SOURCEBOOKS, INC.®
NAPERVILLE, ILLINOIS

Important Note to Readers: This program is intended for healthy adults, age 18 and over. Always consult a medical or health professional before beginning any new diet, nutrition, or exercise program. Neither the author nor the publisher of this book dispense medical advice or prescribe the use of any technique as a form of treatment for physical or medical problems without the advice of a physician, either directly or indirectly. This book is solely for informational and educational purposes and is not medical advice. Individual results may vary.

The intent of the author is only to offer information of a general nature. It is not possible for the author or publisher to know the individual reactions, allergies, etc., of each reader. In all cases, readers must use caution, sample treatments or remedies in small amounts and on inconspicuous test areas, and consult their physicians.

In the event you use any of the information contained in this book for yourself, which is your constitutional right, the author and the publisher assume no responsibility for your actions and do not guarantee individual results.

Published by Sourcebooks, Inc.
P.O. Box 4410, Naperville, Illinois 60567-4410
(630) 961-3900
FAX: (630) 961-2168

Library of Congress Cataloging-in-Publication Data
Irons, Diane
     Diane Irons' 14-day beauty boot camp: the crash course for looking and feeling great / by Diane Irons.
          p. cm.
     Includes index.
     ISBN 1-57071-773-7 (alk. paper)
1. Beauty, Personal. 2. Physical fitness. 3. Diet. I. Title: Diane Irons' fourteen-day beauty boot camp. II. Title: 14-day beauty boot camp. III. Title: Fourteen-day beauty boot camp. IV. Title.

RA778 .I7585 2001
613.7—dc21

                                      2001020074

Printed and bound in the United States of America
DO 10 9 8 7 6 5 4 3 2 1

About the Accompanying CD

This book comes with an audio compact disc containing one track for each day of the Beauty Boot Camp.

The material for each day is intended to be integral to the program, offering advice, tips, and motivation that adds to what you find in the book.

Starting your day with the appropriate track on the CD will serve you best—perhaps you can listen to it when you first wake up, while you shower, or on the way to work. Do your best to make five minutes for it in the morning if you can.

As you listen, keep the book or your journal handy, in case you want to take notes or write down thoughts, feelings, or ideas.

You can certainly use the program in the book by itself and have a terrifically successful Boot Camp makeover. Listening to the accompanying track on the CD, however, will help you get maximum results.

I'm truly honored to be your Boot Camp instructor and give you all my best wishes. I just know you'll be a success!

Diane Irons

TRACK 1	KP Duty
TRACK 2	Set Up for Success
TRACK 3	Basic Training I
TRACK 4	Basic Training II
TRACK 5	Camouflage Camp
TRACK 6	Seize Control
TRACK 7	Reclaiming Self-Value
TRACK 8	Survival Skills
TRACK 9	Daily Diligence
TRACK 10	Self-Defense
TRACK 11	Chemical Warfare
TRACK 12	Budget Boot Camp
TRACK 13	Secret Weapons
TRACK 14	Maintenance Maneuvers

Acknowledgments

My appreciation to the many women and men who have
entrusted me with their faces, figures, and fears.
My love and thanks to my publisher and dear friend, Dominique Raccah,
for her incredible commitment and vision in publishing as well as
her continued support of my work and message.
Kudos to my favorite photographer, Steve Cicco of Boston.
You're there whenever I have a crazy idea, and I never tell you
enough how much I appreciate your wonderful work.
I am overcome with pride over the man my son Kirk has become.
The joy of watching you grow, the privilege of being
your mom, diminishes everything else.
Finally, I can't thank enough, my beloved husband David.
You have been my greatest support, through the joy
and sorrow, and my life's love.

To my dear sisters, Stephanie and Leah.
All my love and gratitude for letting
me experiment on you!

Table of Contents

Introduction

Welcome to my fourteen-day Beauty Boot Camp! This program is about looking better in the quickest way possible. It is derived directly from my life's work in beauty and fitness. After years of working with women of all shapes and sizes, I have consolidated this work into just two weeks. Starting out as a model at the age of thirteen, I was fascinated with how quickly and easily looks could be transformed. I practiced the skills from behind the runways on my friends, sisters, and of course, on myself, while coming up with techniques of my own.

When I am asked to work with a model or celebrity, time is money. My job is to get them into shape, looking fantastic and feeling amazing for the runway, photo shoot, or special appearance. It takes two weeks to accomplish the task of a total makeover. Just fourteen days always gets the job done. We finesse everything from head to toe, including esteem, weight, face, hair, and wardrobe. Now, you can participate in the same program, and in just two weeks you'll see incredible, life-changing results.

The reasons my program has been so successful through the years is that I have made it fun, challenging, and interesting. I have made my plan simple to follow as well as easy to do. Look, life is complicated enough. You don't need to spend hours and hours weighing and measuring your food, applying your makeup, or working out at the gym. And you certainly don't need to spend thousands of dollars collecting the ultimate wardrobe. By making beauty something you can fit into your schedule, I know you're more likely to continue using what you've learned.

Why should we bother with beauty? Why try to create a better, more fit body or a more pulled-together wardrobe? It's a celebration of self. Your appearance is your number one marketing tool. It's the gift you present to the world every single day.

Demonstrating personal pride and style is the ultimate form of self-expression. I believe in letting the person come through, not the designers they're wearing. Nothing you wear should overpower the you that is the artwork. Taking pride in one's appearance is the ultimate act of self-love. And without self-love, it is impossible to give unconditionally to the world.

Your looks should mirror what's inside you. If you have always felt sophisticated, don't try to achieve a cutesy look. It's not going to feel right, and it's not going to wear right on you. We're going to work together to get your body to respond to your needs, not the other way around.

Why do I call my fourteen-day program Beauty Boot Camp? Because for two weeks, there will be no bellyaching, no whining, and no more procrastinating! The reward is that in a very short time, you'll experience results you never thought possible. You're going to learn to become better, and you'll gain more confidence every day. Depending on your goals, you may find that two weeks is all it takes. If you need more time, the drastic improvements you'll see and feel will drive you to the finish line.

You'll be motivated to reach your ultimate goal. Your entire life will change as you continue eating for beauty and health, become more organized, and grow more self-observant.

I'm so excited to share all the secrets of looking and feeling great with you. **_Now let's get to work!_**

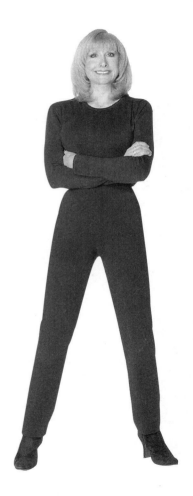

The 14-Day Beauty
Boot Camp Diet

This is the basis of the program, the diet that allows my models to lose anywhere from ten to fifteen pounds while keeping their energy level up and enjoying real food. I've worked with registered dietitian Donna M. De Cunzo, director of nutrition services for eDiets.com, to provide maximum results in the least amount of time, while providing necessary nutrients.

I've chosen and incorporated beauty foods that will have you looking radiant! You'll enjoy the choice of menu, as well as the ease of preparation. You should mix and match the menu items, choosing one for each meal. Each day in this book has a journal page where you should list your choices. Of course, as with any diet, be sure to check with your doctor first for the kind of program and nutrients that are right for you.

This diet is low in sugar and high in protein, complex carbohydrates, and vegetables. You'll eat just three times a day, plus a snack, so that you can discipline your appetite.

Here are some basic rules that underlie the diet. If you do these things everyday, you'll build them as healthy habits that will continue even after you're done with my Beauty Boot Camp.

Water

First and foremost, plan on eight to ten glasses of water daily. Add lots of ice and use fresh lemon or lime to flavor. I suggest following every caffeinated beverage with a glass of ice water to counteract its dehydrating effects. Water regulates body temperature, removes waste products, protects our organs, helps convert food to energy, and cushions our joints. Plus, water will give you a feeling of fullness.

Green Tea

Try to acquire a taste for green tea, which is filled with valuable antioxidants. It's also important for its metabolic burning effects. Try to drink three cups a day.

Don't Eat After 8 P.M.

Unless you can only eat your dinner at or after this time, make 8 P.M. the shutdown time for your kitchen. Try not to eat for at least three hours before bedtime, if possible. Eating in the evening often leads to over-consumption of unneeded calories. You'll find yourself more alert and ready to go in the morning. Plus, you may be more willing to consume the most important meal of the day—breakfast.

Go for Fiber

Foods with a high fiber content are natural appetite suppressants, since they take up more room in your stomach than other foods. Fiber is also slower to digest, so it keeps hunger away for a longer period of time. A recent U.S. Department of Agriculture study found that for each gram of fiber you consume, you absorb seven fewer calories from food. This is because most fiber leaves the body undigested.

Breakfast

Choose One

#1

1 cup bran flakes or any other high fiber cereal
⅔ cup wild blueberries
1 cup nonfat milk or soy milk
coffee/tea
ice water

#2

2 eggs, scrambled in a nonstick pan or microwaved,
    and seasoned with pepper and parsley
1 cup spinach
salsa
coffee/tea
ice water

#3

1 Breakfast Melt made with 1 small pita pocket,
    ½ cup cottage or ricotta cheese, and cinnamon
    to taste; spread cheese over pita, top with cinnamon,
    and broil until bubbling
coffee/tea
ice water

#4

1 cup hot cereal, such as oat bran
⅔ cup strawberries
1 cup nonfat milk or soy milk
coffee/tea
ice water

#5

2 fat-free waffles
¼ cup sugar-free syrup
1 small nonfat yogurt
coffee/tea
ice water

Lunch
Choose One

#1
Pizza made with ½ pita pocket, 1 ounce shredded mozzarella cheese, 1 tomato, oregano, garlic powder, Italian seasoning, and pepper to taste

Salad of mixed greens, carrots, tomatoes, and celery with 2 Tbsp. of fat-free dressing or balsamic vinegar

coffee/tea

ice water

#2
Turkey sandwich made with 3 slices roasted turkey, ½ pita pocket and mustard

Salad of mixed greens, carrots, tomatoes, and celery with 2 Tbsp. of fat-free dressing or balsamic vinegar

coffee/tea

ice water

#3
Tuna sandwich made with 2 slices of 40 calorie wheat bread, albacore tuna packed in water, fat-free mayo, and spices

Salad of mixed greens, carrots, tomatoes and celery with 2 Tbsp. of fat-free dressing or balsamic vinegar

coffee/tea

ice water

#4
Vegetable tortilla made with 1 flour tortilla, ½ cup reduced-fat shredded Monterey Jack cheese, shredded lettuce, ½ cup diced zucchini, and ¼ cup diced red pepper; fill tortilla and broil

Salad of mixed greens, carrots, tomatoes, and celery with 2 Tbsp. of fat-free dressing or balsamic vinegar

coffee/tea

ice water

#5
Grilled cheese sandwich made with 1½ ounces low-fat or soy cheese and tomatoes on 2 slices of wheat bread

Salad of mixed greens, carrots, tomatoes, and celery with 2 Tbsp. of fat-free dressing or balsamic vinegar

coffee/tea

ice water

Dinner
Choose One

#1

4 ounces chicken or fish, broiled

2 cups cooked vegetables, drizzled with lemon

1 small baked potato, topped with 1 tsp. plain yogurt

coffee/tea

ice water

#2

chicken salad made with 3 ounces chicken, ½ cup cooked pasta, 2 Tbsp. low-fat mayonnaise, shredded lettuce, tomato, celery, shredded carrots, and onion

coffee/tea

ice water

#3

Baked scallops made with ¼ pound scallops, 1 Tbsp. white wine or apple juice, lemon to taste; baked at 400 degrees for 20 minutes or microwaved for 6 minutes

coffee/tea

ice water

#4

Turkey fajitas made with a 6" tortilla, 3 ounces skinless turkey breast, stir-fried bell pepper and onion cooked using cooking spray, and ½ ounce low-fat cheddar cheese

coffee/tea

ice water

#5

Soy burger on a small whole wheat roll

Salad of mixed greens, carrots, tomatoes, and celery with 2 Tbsp. of fat-free dressing or balsamic vinegar

coffee/tea

ice water

Snack
Choose One

#1
an apple and 2 Tbsp. of reduced-fat peanut butter

#2
1 cup watermelon

#3
½ cup nonfat frozen yogurt

#4
8 ounces of nonfat yogurt

#5
2 cups of air-popped popcorn

KP Duty

Today is the first day on the road to success and the makeover where you learn by doing. It's fun to watch those makeovers on talk shows. I've been on these shows myself, orchestrating looks that allow the participant to look thinner, sexier, younger...you name it I've done it. It demonstrates to the participant and the audience the untapped possibilities and potential that lie within. The problem is that the person who is being made over is not learning how to do it.

They have makeup artists, wardrobe stylists, and hair masters performing the transformation for them. So how are they going to maintain that look? Are they going to take these people home with them? Of course not! That's why it's so important that you do the work, not just sit there and try to absorb it all.

Your life and your looks are about to change. Here in Day One of Beauty Boot Camp, we're cleaning out. It may sound like an odd way to start, but it is so important, because it provides organization as well as a foundation to work from. It's the day you level the playing field and clean out the clutter that is not allowing you to go forth and be what you want to be, to have the body and the mind set that will allow you to look just the way you've always imagined.

It is absolutely necessary to go through everything in your daily routine and remove the clutter. There's lots of toxic stuff in your environment, and I'm here to help you to detoxify the elements while you clean out your body and psyche.

Water, Water, Everywhere

The first component of this program and a thread that you'll see throughout it is the importance of water. In order for you to truly realize your success, right now you need to commit to drinking at least eight to ten glasses of water a day.

Water is the number one makeover secret, and one you must employ. Drinking water is important for keeping the skin hydrated, decreasing hunger, regulating body temperature, removing wastes, and protecting our organs. Water helps convert food to energy, and it cushions our joints.

CLEAN

OUT

THE

CLUTTER

IN

YOUR

MIND,

BODY,

AND

CLOSET.

When models or legendary beauties are asked to share their absolute favorite beauty secret, they'll often say "drinking lots of water." That means they really don't want you to know their secret. You see, these lovelies are only sharing half the story. It's drinking *ice cold* water that keeps them looking their best.

With each glass of ice water you drink, your body has to heat itself up in order to be able to accept the ice, since the body's normal temperature is 98.6 degrees. This act fuels up the body, firing up the metabolism. It's the only case of the phrase "negative calories" having any merit. With each glass that you drink, your body will expend up to twenty-five calories.

By drinking up to ten eight-ounce glasses of water a day, you will not only increase your metabolic rate, but you'll burn as much as 250 extra calories. Compare that to your treadmill or stair-stepper! If you find it difficult to get that much water down, flavor it with fresh lemon or lime to make it more palatable and refreshing. An easy way to carry water is to freeze a couple of bottles and pack them with you. They'll slowly defrost as you go through your day.

Cleaning the Clutter

It's vital to get rid of all the extra stuff that is literally and emotionally weighing you down. Today, go through each room of your house and pack up the stuff you don't need or use. Have no mercy!

First, let's check out your kitchen. Go through each cabinet and organize it in such a way that the good foods and staples are easily located. Throw away all the junk foods that you can, and stick the rest out of sight. Who needs the temptation? Also, if you can store items in portion sizes, do that now. It will lessen the chance of second-guessing your serving size and subsequently over- or undereating.

Check out the refrigerator, and toss all the frozen candy bars and unbearably gross, fake, fat foods. If you need to keep anything you shouldn't be eating, hide it under aluminum foil. Label it in the least descriptive manner possible. For instance, if you need to store brownies in the fridge, label them as "brownies," not "double fudge brownies." The written word can easily tempt us off track.

Next, head to your closet for some heavy duty pitching. Get rid of anything that doesn't look smashing on you, and I don't care how much you paid for it. Even expensive clothing gets tired and needs to be put to rest. If you haven't worn it in two years, say goodbye! Toss anything that has permanent holes or stains. A trend that never made it to classic status is now dead, and you need to bury it!

There are things that may be in your closet that keep popping back as trends, but never should have been in style to begin with. Say good bye to stirrup pants, slogan tee shirts, decorated sweatshirts, and those stupid pleated skirts that make even the slimmest models look hippy.

Your bathroom needs to be both cleaned out and turned into a home spa. It will become a refuge where you'll do some of

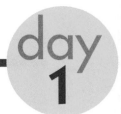

your finest work. There should be nothing in your bathroom that will not enhance your beauty and allow you to accurately make personal assessments.

In your cosmetic bag, get rid of any unflattering shades and colors that are not perfectly matched to your skin tones. Bring a mirror to outside lighting to evaluate your colors. Toss eye shadows over twelve months old, any cosmetic that has an odor, cosmetics that separate, as well as mascara more than four months old. Get rid of applicators older than three months if they can't be shampooed or washed with soap and water.

Next, in your medicine cabinet, it's important that you keep only the freshest vitamins. You want to ensure that they're providing the nutrients you need during Beauty Boot Camp. There's an easy way (besides the expiration date) to tell if they're fresh or not. Put one in a bowl of vinegar for thirty minutes. If it hasn't dissolved, then the vitamin or supplement should be thrown out. If they can't dissolve in the vinegar, then they won't emulsify in your body and do their job.

Be sure to check your hair dryer. If it doesn't have the power it used to, its air vents may need to be cleaned. Unplug the dryer, then use a tweezer and an old toothbrush to remove any hair and lint. Now's the time to clean your brushes, combs, and Velcro rollers. A lint brush can be used to take the hair that's stuck and twisted on the rollers.

Cleaning Out You

While you're cleaning out all around you, now is the time to learn to clean out your body with an easy deep breathing exercise. Your body needs oxygen, and breathing in a measured, thoughtful way will give you a vehicle to connect with your inner self. Take a long full breath. Really fill up your lungs. Make sure that you relax your with each exhalation.

Today's cleaning out will reduce your regime to its downright simplicity. It's key to clean and organize yourself so nothing will break your stride.

You should be feeling relaxed, refreshed, and ready to go. There's something about a good cleansing that just melts the stress away.

So today, Day One of Beauty Boot Camp, set yourself up for success. Get to cleaning out that clutter in your home, your body, and your mind, and come back and see me tomorrow. We're on the road to a new you—and you can do it!

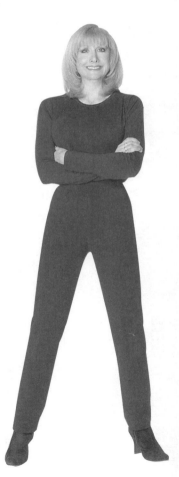

Diane's Tips:

EXTRA
Cleaning Tips

1 It's most important to check how you're cleaning while you're cleaning out. If you are washing your face with soap every morning, not only are you wasting your time, but you're needlessly drying out your skin. If you've properly cleansed your face the evening before, your moisturizer should still be doing its job. All you need to do is to remove the excess oils and reactivate the moisturizer's film with a splash of water.

2 If your skin is extremely oily, just mix a bit of powdered milk with enough water to make a paste. Apply briefly, then rinse. It will gently remove the oils. I learned this from French models who keep charming potpourri jars filled with powdered milk by their sink basins. They wouldn't dream of using the soap they use to wash their hands and bodies on their lovely faces.

On the **MAGAZINE** Rack

Magazines with computer or otherwise altered images won't help you achieve your goal, so they need to go. Here's what you really need to know in order to understand why they may be sabotaging your efforts—even the models don't look like they do in some of those photographs. Our bodies have been stretched out and air brushed. I even remember remarking to a photographer that I didn't realize my legs were so long. "They're not," he shot back sarcastically, "they've been stretched." *Oh the pain!*

Look, if you've never weighed 110 pounds, your body is probably not programmed to be at such a low weight. You might be able to get there by pure grit and deprivation, but you won't be able to maintain that weight. Trying to stay there will affect your health, your looks, and may lead to eating disorders. You can copy celebrity techniques, but you can only remain YOU—and there's so much of YOU to discover.

My Journal:

Write three goals you hope to accomplish in this program.

1. _Weight 110_
2. _Better skin_
3. _____

List three habits you need to break (for example, nail biting, chocolate addiction, etc.)

1. _Snacking after work_
2. _Skipping meals_
3. _____

List what you threw out today and reflect on how it made you feel.

_____

_____

What is one routine in your day that is too cumbersome?

Keeping up ō laundry

_____

_____

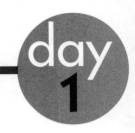
day 1

If you got rid of it, what would you do with the extra time?

Special projects

List eight times in your typical day when it will be easiest to fit in those all-important glasses of ice water.

1st thing in Am
Drive to work
Meetings
Lunch
Drive home
Dinner
Bedtime

"In fourteen days, I want to feel _thinner_ !"

Weight
_____

Waist
_____

Hips
_____

Bust
_____

Thighs
_____

Boot Camp Basics:

Care and Maintenance

After spending precious dollars on your wardrobe, shoes, and accessories, it makes sense to keep them in top condition. They'll last longer and be ready for you at a moment's notice.

☑ Wrap hangers in tissue paper to support heavy clothing.

☐ Keep leather garments and shoes supple by treating them with protective cream.

☑ Iron clothes inside out to avoid dulling the fabric's finish.

☐ When storing clothes, keep moths away by placing dry bay leaves between layers in storage boxes and garment bags. Bay leaves won't leave the unpleasant odor of mothballs.

☐ Apply a thin coat of clear nail polish or nail hardener on pearl buttons to restore their luster and make them more durable.

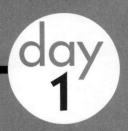

❑ Rub clothing with ammonia before laundering to remove deodorant stains.

❑ Perfume padded hangers to scent clothing.

❑ To remove salt stains from shoes and boots, blot with white vinegar.

❑ Erase dark marks from pale leather by dabbing with nail polish remover.

❑ Clean patent leather with glass cleaner.

❑ Install a hook on the outside of your closet door. Use it to air out the clothing you've worn that day before returning it to the closet. This saves money on dry cleaning.

❑ Stuff boots with old magazines to retain their shape.

day one
my diet today

Breakfast: _____

_____

Lunch: _____

_____

Dinner: _____

_____

Snack: _____

_____

Glasses of Water:

☐ ☐ ☐ ☐ ☐ ☐ ☐ ☐ ☐ ☐

Set Up for Success

day
2

PREPARE

YOUR

LIFE

FOR

SUCCESSFUL

CHANGES.

You've cleaned out on Day One, and now it's time to set up shop. To set the scene for success, you should surround yourself with your favorite things. Think about what makes you feel great. Think about what makes you feel most attractive.

Set Your Bedroom Scene

During this program you should do all you can to get at least nine hours of sleep. You'll run out of gas quickly if you don't, plus I want you to get into the habit of sleeping for beauty and health. More importantly, if you don't make a commitment to get this added rest, you'll be tempted to shore up your energy with food. If you set up your bedroom properly, it will become a welcome retreat.

To get your sleep, you need to put your entire bedroom in the mood! Your bedroom should become more desirable than your kitchen.

Make sure your bedroom becomes pitch black with the shades drawn. Avoid even the light from a digital clock. I'd also like for you to soften the lighting throughout your sleeping quarters, including your reading lamps. Reading here should be like a lullaby, just enough to put you to sleep.

Set Up Your Closet

Organizing your closet should be done in a way that will allow you to get ready at a moment's notice.

A great way to organize is to hang your clothing by both color and function. The easiest way to dress quickly is to pre-coordinate entire outfits, including belts and jewelry. They're ready to go and so are you, pulled together with style and panache.

Organize your earrings and pins by hanging them from the belt of your garments. If you need a garment bag, cut a small opening in a pillowcase. Don't ever buy garment bags made from plastic, because they don't allow your fabrics to breathe.

Group together daytime apparel, weekend wear, and special occasion outfits. Although you certainly can mix and match for the right occasion, for efficiency, this is the easiest approach. Here's a hint: I like to use different colored shower curtain rings to separate categories of clothing.

Mirrors

If you've ever visited a spa, then you've seen that there are mirrors at every nook and cranny. If you're looking for an accurate evaluation, who will be more honest than you? Try to place a mirror in every room as a continual checkpoint for your looks. It's an indicator of what needs to be finessed, as well as just what the world will see.

The most important spot in your home for a mirror is probably the oddest. You need at least one in the kitchen, and you need a magnetic mirror on your refrigerator. They're sold at most drugstores and mass merchandise outlets. If you have to face yourself each time you start to open the fridge door, it will remind you better than any picture or slogan could of your goals. Don't forget to smile when you pass it by!

Setting Up Your Cosmetics

Your makeup center will become your private sanctuary. It should be streamlined and minimized to be both highly functional and time-efficient. I encourage you to find some of the great products that perform more than one job. In drugstores, you'll find foundations that function as both concealer and powder. You'll find them called "cream to powder," "all in one," or "two way" foundations. What I particularly like about them is that not only do they eliminate the need for powder, but the coverage is also quite forgiving. It's great to carry with you because it can be applied during the day as a touch-up. Look for oil-free formulas for the longest lasting coverage.

Eye shadow can double as a soft eyeliner, and it provides a natural look. You may find that you prefer shading your eyes this way, both because of the time-saving factor (its application doesn't require great precision or a steady hand), and because there's not so much pulling at the tender eye tissue.

Bathroom Set Up

Keep a scale and tape measure handy for accurate assessment. Although it's important to weigh yourself daily, it's not the only indication that you're getting in shape. The amount of water you've had in the last few hours, the salt in your food, etc., can make a difference in your weight. Even though it's only "water weight," it can be disconcerting. Take your measurements each day, as you weigh yourself, to mark your progress.

Keep something you're dying to fit into on the bathroom door. Make sure it's in sight, and if you can, try it on every few days. It could be a pair of jeans, a bathing suit, or a dress you're trying to get into. Even if it won't go over your hips, each effort will keep you from letting up. It should become easier with each attempt.

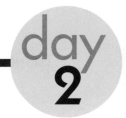

Start Your Journal

If you've never successfully kept a journal before, I'm asking you to really give it a shot now. Look, it's only for two weeks, and it will tell you so much. You saw that Day One in this book included space for journal entries. You may wish to also keep a separate journal allowing you more space to write. The first entry might start out including your goals and the reasons for getting there.

Another valuable entry is how you feel your life will change when you reach your goal, or at least how you expect it to be different. Also include the action plan that will get you there. List your strategy. It can be as simple as walking instead of taking the elevator. When you do feel yourself slipping up, putting those thoughts down in your journal will help you understand the nature of your behavior.

Create a Home Spa

The most effective beauty routines can be done in the privacy of your own home. You can create your own personal spa, and at the end of the day there is nothing quite so wonderful! It needs to be properly set up so that everything is on hand and waiting for you to perform your magic. I like to use a small laundry basket to keep everything in one place.

You should include a loofah or a coarse washcloth for exfoliating your body and for increasing the detox benefits of your spa. A simple dry brushing takes only a few minutes and is an effective way of stimulating the lymphatic system. It gives the skin a healthy glow and breaks down cellulite. Dry brushing is done in the top spas and is one of the nicest parts of Beauty Boot Camp. A foot file or pumice will also work on knees, heels, and elbows. Get one that can be washed and sanitized.

Scents, oils, and candles can relieve all the stress that's been building up during the day and give you the atmosphere that will take you to a different place. You can also use oils in the bath, as a massage, and as a room spray. You'll find a treasure trove, attractively priced, at most natural supermarkets and health food stores. Even vanilla and almond food extracts can lift your mood and spirit.

Here's another water alert. Sip lots of it during your spa treatments to aid hydration. Also, apply your moisturizer while bathing to enhance its benefits.

Don't worry, it sounds like it's a lot to do, but once it becomes routine, you'll go through your treatments with pure joy and anticipation. All the benefits that you'll quickly see and feel will put to rest any thought of cutting corners.

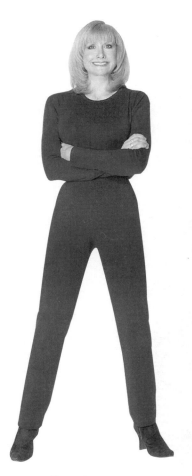

Diane's Tips:

TOOL TIME

All you really need are a few select beauty tools. They will make all the difference in creating a polished, stylish appearance. You don't need to spend a lot of money on them. I love to shop in the art supply departments of mass merchandise stores for my brushes. The quality is excellent, and there's always a good selection.

You'll need a **vent brush**. Its teeth vary in height and are spaced far apart. This creates a lifting action and will help your hair dry faster. A **paddle brush** straightens and smoothes hair so it's less likely to frizz. A paddle brush will allow you to do two- to three-inch sections at a time.

If you need curve and curl in your hair, a **metal round brush** is a sound investment. This brush takes the place of a curling iron and is less damaging to hair. Styles can be virtually "locked in" with a final blast of cold air.

Velcro rollers allow hair to set and form after it is blown dry. The larger the roller, the straighter the style. If you want to get an assortment of different sizes, purchase two jumbo, two extra large, two large, and four medium. That should be enough for any style.

Start your makeup brush collection with a **big fluffy brush** for applying blush and loose powder. Test it to make sure that it is soft, yet compact. One **eye shadow brush** is all you'll need. It should be small and rounded for blending and contouring the eye area.

A **lip brush**, although not necessary, is great for blending colors and applying definitive lines. Try to find one with a slightly pointed brush.

If you have room, include a **large blusher**. It allows powder to appear more natural, and will glide over lines. Just a spritz of hairspray will keep the powder on the brush.

My Journal:

What changes have you made in your environment today? You should try to make at least five.

1. _____
2. _____
3. _____
4. _____
5. _____

List a spa treatment you'd like to try. Post a reminder to yourself in your bathroom.

_____
_____
_____

Name three high stress points of your day and the events surrounding them. Think about how you dealt with each one of them. Did you handle it well? How could you have handled it better?

1. _____
_____
_____

2. _____

_____

_____

3. _____

_____

_____

Finish the following sentence with three things that you like about yourself. "When I look in the mirror, I see…"

1. _____
2. _____
3. _____

Boot Camp Basics:

Destressing Basics

A home spa provides the most important beauty routines. The body is often affected by stress even before the mind has registered it. Learn to relax while looking better with these treatments.

☑ Orange Juice Bath: The vitamin C in this bath will revitalize and rejuvenate your skin. Cut oranges up and place them in a warm bath. Soak for twenty minutes.

☐ Add two teaspoons dried lavender mixed with one teaspoon of lavender oil to a filled tub. Lavender's relaxing fragrance relaxes the body and aids sleep.

☐ Combine one teaspoon olive oil with the contents of a vitamin E capsule. Massage into your hands and slip on a pair of cotton gloves. Wear overnight.

☐ Treat dandruff with one teaspoon jojoba oil and five drops of tea tree oil combined. Dab on scalp and let set for thirty minutes.

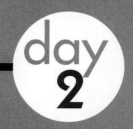

☐ Soothe your muscles by applying a thin film of bath oil over your shoulders and neck. Drape a large towel over your shoulders and step into the shower. The towel's wet heat will help the oil penetrate, softening skin and relaxing muscles.

☐ Honey and Yogurt Body Treatment: Combine two cups plain yogurt with two teaspoons honey. Apply over body and let soak in for five minutes. Rinse off. This treatment conditions, cleanses, and moisturizes.

☐ Condition oily hair with the juice of one lemon mixed with 1/4 cup cider vinegar. Use it as a final rinse.

☐ Give yourself a hot stone massage for at-home reflexology. Pick the smoothest rocks you can find and boil them to a very warm, yet comfortable temperature. Place them on the back of your neck, in between your toes, and wherever you're feeling tense.

☐ Add a splash of raspberry vinegar to your bath for extra skin softening.

day two

my diet today

Breakfast: _____

_____

Lunch: _____

_____

Dinner: _____

_____

Snack: _____

_____

Glasses of Water:

☐ ☐ ☐ ☐ ☐ ☐ ☐ ☐ ☐ ☐

Basic Training I

LEARN

THE

BASIC

SKILLS

OF

THE

BEAUTY

MASTERS.

Beauty Boot Camp begins from the very moment you open your eyes. If you're like so many of your Boot Camp buddies, you are desperate for coffee in the morning. Try to hold off until you drink a glass of ice water to stoke your metabolism.

Get in the habit of drinking a glass of ice water before each meal. Foods with high water content are also beneficial in helping you to feel fuller and, subsequently, to eat less. Be sure to have lots of tomatoes, grapes, and apples on hand to help assuage your appetite throughout the day.

Check your weight without clothing or jewelry, and take your waist measurement. Write both down in your journal.

Start your morning with your favorite upbeat music. Use it to keep yourself moving as you go through your routines. While you're brushing your teeth, don't just stand there—here's your chance to start exercising! Dance, perform side lunges, and lift your legs back and high for extra butt firming.

In this program, you must make time to eat a complete breakfast. You'll be less hungry at lunch, have more energy, and be more creative for your effort. Set your alarm to get up fifteen minutes earlier if necessary. Preprogram your coffeemaker, set the table, do whatever's necessary to include this basic morning ritual. It will provide you with the strength and commitment to face the rest of your day.

Basic Training Smile

The basis of any great smile is white teeth. When you brush, be sure you are brushing both your teeth and your tongue. It sounds like such a basic step, and yet so many people either forget this step or pay for expensive tongue scrapers. You're not through brushing until you've brushed that coating off of your tongue.

You need to add this technique to your basic skills, so that you not only remove bacteria but the coating that causes bad breath and the unpleasant sensation that may lead to overeating. If you find yourself eating when you're not even hungry, you might be attempting to eat off that coating with food.

Learn to brush your teeth and tongue the right way. Always apply toothpaste to a dry brush. Brush up and down for at least two minutes. It takes that long to remove plaque. Studies have shown that most of us brush sideways and for less than a minute.

Basic Training Face

The way you prepare your skin in the morning will make all the difference in how your makeup looks, and how long it lasts. There's a different regime for each skin type.

Dry: Dry skin has a fine texture with small pores. It often feels "tight" or "pulled," and it is prone to broken capillaries. Don't bother with cleansing your skin in the morning. Your skin needs only a splash of water to remove excess oils. You really don't need to bother with a toner, but if your face just doesn't feel clean without this step, witch hazel is inexpensive and much preferred over toners containing alcohol. Follow with a rich moisturizer and wait for a minute or two before applying your makeup to allow the moisturizer to be absorbed into the skin.

Oily: Signs of oily skin are actual oil "spots," especially prominent on the nose, forehead, and chin. The pores of the skin are large and visible to the eye. Don't be overly aggressive, as you may be tempted to be, to treat this type of skin. The best cleanser is powdered milk mixed with water, which is both a lactic acid wash and exfoliant. You'll not only cleanse the skin, but you'll also get rid of surface debris and oils. Restore the pH balance with a mix of equal amounts of lemon juice and water. Although it may not seem necessary to use moisturizer at all, you should use an oil-free moisturizer right under your eyes.

Combination: This type of skin is actually a combination of oily skin in the T-zone of the face (nose, forehead, and chin) and dry skin everywhere else. Again, use powdered milk, but only in the oily areas, and follow up with witch hazel toner, concentrating on the T-zone area. An oil-free gel or moisturizer is the perfect surface to allow your makeup to go over smoothly.

Basic Training Makeup

Putting on makeup is a skill that should never take more than ten minutes of your day. Many of the great beauties I've worked with have used this time as a form of meditation. And it makes such perfect sense. After all, you're touching your face, you're gazing into the mirror. It is the perfect opportunity to center yourself for the day. Scheduling these ten minutes in is an integral part of Beauty Boot Camp. It will get your day off to a great start!

1. Apply foundation with your fingers or a sponge. I prefer to use my fingers when I'm looking for a more "natural" appearance. The warmth of your fingers will allow your foundation to spread more quickly and evenly. This method also provides you with more control over the coverage. Always start at the under-eye area. This is where coverage is most important. Pat gently into the area. Never pull anywhere near the eye—the eye tissue is delicate and you don't want to cause unnecessary wrinkling.

2. "Lift" your eye and frame your face with a few strokes to the eyebrow. Use a toothbrush or old washed mascara wand sprayed with a bit of hair gel. Dip an eyeliner brush into an eye shadow closest to your brow color if you need to fill in. If eyes are

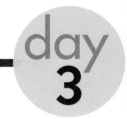

the windows to the soul, then the eyebrows are the valances. They have the ability to change facial expressions and take away years. The basic skill of eyebrow design is worth developing.

3. Brush a neutral eye shadow over the entire lid. Deepen the color in the crease and slightly above the outer corner of the eye. Use a kohl pencil or darker shadow around the eye, and smudge a bit to eliminate any harsh, unnatural lines. Curl your lashes, and lightly coat with mascara. Hold your eye "up" while you're doing this by placing your finger at the arch of your brow

4. Use a neutral lip pencil over moistened lips (use balm or moisturizer first).

5. Dab off a bit of that lip color with your finger and lightly blend over the apples of your cheeks for a natural, coordinating blush.

6. Finish your look by contouring with bronzing powder at your cheekbones, under your jaw line, and down the side of your nose. Remember that basic blush application begins at the apple of the cheek. From there, work in a light circular motion towards the upper cheekbone.

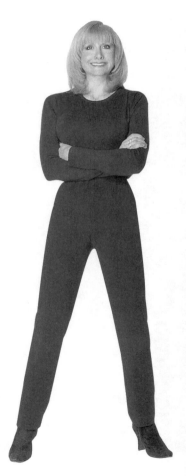

Basic Training Eating

To get through Beauty Boot Camp, there are basics you need to have on hand, ready to go at a moment's notice. You'll rely on these staples to keep you away from temptation. Read labels to make basic low-fat choices. Be prepared by keeping the flavor while cutting the calories. Sweeten fruit with cinnamon, flavor your water, and treat yourself to quality foods.

Buy vegetables that are already cleaned and chopped for you. Frozen vegetables can be microwaved right in the box in a matter of minutes. Look in the meat department for preportioned sizes of chicken, beef, and fish.

There are so many convenience foods in your supermarkets, you just have to stock your kitchen with the right ammunition for success.

Basic Training Posture

Ten-hut! Here's an easy way to keep your back straight. Keep your chin elevated, and try to push your shoulder blades together. Remember to check your posture throughout the day.

Now look in your mirror to check your basic beauty looks. Does your skin look smooth and fresh? Does your makeup enhance your looks? Go face the world with your beautiful looks!

Diane's Tips:

BASIC TRAINING BRA

The foundation of your wardrobe lies within.

Unless you're wearing the right undergarments, your clothing won't do you justice. Yet, eight out of ten women are wearing the wrong size bra, and it's usually too small. This leads to bulges, lack of support, and a sloppy look no matter what you're wearing.

Here's how to measure: while wearing a bra, pull a tape measure around your torso below your breasts and add one inch. Round up if you get an odd number like thirty-five. This is your band size. Find your cup size by pulling the tape measure firmly around the fullest part of your bust. Then subtract the first number (the band size) from your cup size.

A one-inch difference equates to an A cup.
Two inches is a B cup,
up to three inches is a C cup,
up to four inches is a D cup, and
up to five inches a double D cup.

With each weight change of ten pounds or more, you should take this measurement again.

How can you tell if your bra fits properly?

The center seam should lie flat against your breastbone without any gaps between cups. The back band should hit just below your shoulder blades. The front band should be loose enough to run your finger underneath, and your bra should be perfectly comfortable when it's hooked on the middle row of hooks.

A beige bra should be your basic color choice, since it doesn't show through your clothing as much as white or other colors. If you're a woman of color, then choose a taupe color, never black. If your breasts are uneven, a stretchy bra will allow for that difference. Any wrinkling in the bra means that your bra's cup size is too large. Any bulging means that the cup is too small.

No matter what your bust size, it's always necessary to wear a bra. Your bust tissue will break down if you don't, causing sagging and stretch marks.

My Journal:

What are the physical changes you want to make in your looks in this program and beyond? List as many as you can. Remember to keep your goals measurable and attainable.

_____
_____
_____
_____
_____
_____
_____
_____
_____
_____
_____
_____
_____

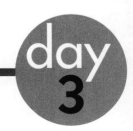

Describe your mindset toward your looks and how it could change for the better.

_____

_____

_____

_____

_____

_____

Write one goal for tomorrow and how you plan to achieve it. Tomorrow, be sure to read this goal again as soon as you get up in the morning.

_____

_____

_____

_____

_____

Skin Basics

Keep these skin basics at home. The best moisturizers and toners are no further than your grocery or health food store.

- ☑ Almond oil is excellent for all skin types to soften and smooth skin. It's also helpful in relieving itching, irritation, and inflammation.

- ☐ Apply aloe vera gel as a toner. It contains healing properties that renew cells, and it is gentle on the skin.

- ☐ Apricot kernel oil is good for delicate and mature skins. It's extremely rich in vitamin A and should be applied to wrinkled and extremely dry skin.

- ☐ Use cocoa butter to smooth out scars.

- ☐ Combine kosher salt with safflower oil to exfoliate your face and body.

- ☐ Flaxseed oil is useful in promoting cell regeneration. Use it for treating stretch marks.

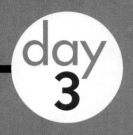

day
3

☐ Remove blackheads by combining 1/4 cup boiling water with one teaspoon Epsom salts and three drops of iodine. Let the mixture cool until it's comfortable to the touch. To loosen blackheads, dab it on with a cotton ball.

☐ Massage a small amount of honey all over your face. Let it set for about ten minutes. Remove with a cotton ball dipped in grapefruit juice. Leave juice on five minutes before rinsing with warm water.

☐ Mix one packet powdered laxative and two cups of boiling water in a large bowl. Use it to clean and steam out impurities by placing your face as close to the bowl as comfortable.

☐ Massage away dry skin with one tablespoon dried kelp combined with one tablespoon vegetable shortening. Massage into skin with a coarse cloth or toothbrush and wipe off.

my diet today

Breakfast: _____

_____

Lunch: _____

_____

Dinner: _____

_____

Snack: _____

_____

Glasses of Water:

☐ ☐ ☐ ☐ ☐ ☐ ☐ ☐ ☐ ☐

Basic Training II

MASTER TIME- AND MONEY-SAVING SKILLS.

Today is day two of Basic Training. We're looking to master skills that you'll use throughout the rest of Beauty Boot Camp and beyond. Through practice and perseverance, these skills will become habitual, practically second nature, meaning you'll achieve a better look in less time and with less frustration.

Food Mastery

In order to become the master of your body and feel in control on a daily basis, it's important to have a daily game plan.

Find restaurants and fast-food outlets that offer calorie counts and low-fat alternatives. If there's no choice, take control of the menu by asking that your dressings and spreads be served on the side. You should always be prepared to come up with an alternative plan on the spot, because life is never a straight line when it comes to diet.

Check the calorie counts of what you eat. Many people watch only the number of fat grams, and this is a big mistake. To calculate the maximum calories you can consume and still be able to lose weight, simply add a zero to your current weight. For example, someone who weighs 140 pounds can have up to 1,400 calories a day and still lose weight.

I've purposely not given you a great variety of foods to choose from in the Beauty Boot Camp diet. Not only do I not want you to have to think too much about what you're eating, but studies have shown that the more food choices we have, the more we will eat.

Master your cravings by visualizing how you'll look in clothes that fit and flatter. Think about all the energy you'll have and how you'll be able to participate in more activities. It brings food right back into place, doesn't it?

Grocery shop with a list, and you'll be less likely to compulsively pick out foods that are not on your program. Without an exact list, not only will you end up with items that will take you off track, but you'll spend up to a third more than shoppers with a list.

Makeup Mastery

Mastering makeup techniques will make all the difference between looking like you've covered yourself with war paint and giving the illusion that you've been naturally blessed. The method by which you apply makeup is more important than the type of makeup you use, or its price point. Although I'm happy to teach you the top secrets of the industry, it's your own practicing in front of the mirror that will provide you with the expertise. Try to make time to experiment with new looks.

Foundation is always the mainstay of a great look. Nobody's face is flawless, and you need to provide your face with uniformity. That's why I don't believe in applying foundation to only parts of the face, as some artists recommend. It never looks right because there's no absolutely perfect color match. If you really want your face to have a natural finish, take a bit of moisturizer and add it to your foundation. The amount you use will dictate whether you are applying a light foundation or a tinted moisturizer.

When you become a makeup master, you can stretch out your cosmetics, and streamline your product line. Eye shadows can be used to color-correct skin tones and imperfections. Yellow eye shadow added to a bit of foundation conceals dark circles. Blue eye shadow added to foundation gets rid of ruddy tones and broken capillaries.

Often when I'm working with an older client, powdery shadows and blushes tend to look too chalky, exaggerating wrinkling. A little bit of baby oil blended into these powders creates a creamy consistency. It's a myth that only the very young can wear shine. Too much matte ages the face, while shine illuminates it.

Facial contouring is a skill that scares everyone because it can look extremely garish if done incorrectly. The easiest way to contour is with a foundation shade that is no more than two shades darker than your actual facial skin tone. Tap it very lightly down the sides of your nose, under the cheekbones, under the chin and jaw line, and on the tip of the nose if it needs shortening. Start out with cream for ease of blending, and then move on to bronzing powder for lasting coverage.

After applying lipstick, add a little light eye shadow to the upper and lower center of the lip. Blend slightly for a pouty effect. If you have large lips, don't bother with liner. To achieve a less defined look, soften the edge with your finger or a cotton swab. For thin lips, draw slightly beyond the lip with a neutral pencil. Then apply your lipstick. It will adhere to the liner.

After your makeup application, take apart a tissue and dab it all over your face. It blends the makeup together and softens your look.

Skin Mastery

Wouldn't it be great to have skin that you want to show off, rather than cover up? It can be achieved! You can master this, your largest organ, with a little work and pampering. Here's my water alert again. I usually can tell who's been drinking enough water. Their skin is clearer and has an actual glow to it. Drinking water and getting enough rest are probably the top two secrets to great skin.

Diet is the most important element of skin care. Although it's an old wives tale that eating chocolate causes pimples, you really can feed your skin internally by eating fresh, less processed foods. So eat what you want your skin to wear. Would you rather look like the results of a fresh peach or a salted potato chip? You'll be amazed at how quickly small changes in your diet can help in your overall appearance.

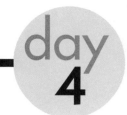

You need to feed and control your skin topically as well. Limit sun exposure, and be sure to wear sunscreen whenever you're outside. Keep your hands away from your face. Hands carry germs that are often transferred to our faces. Exercise also helps flush impurities out of the skin.

Master the use of vitamins as a fresh additive to basic moisturizers. If you're fighting wrinkles, break open a vitamin A capsule and add it to a thimbleful of a basic drugstore moisturizer. Extra dryness can easily be treated by adding a vitamin E capsule to enough moisturizer to make it spreadable but not slippery.

Be aware of your environment. You may want to add a humidifier to your house if it gets very dry. Wash off the mouthpiece of your phone weekly. It could cause chin breakouts. If you wear glasses, including sunglasses, clean them with rubbing alcohol. Take care of your skin and be diligent about it. Finding what works for your particular skin type takes time and patience. When you do, the results will be magnificent.

Hair Mastery

Unless your hair's working, nothing else will. No matter how hard you try, your look just won't come together. Although everyone's hair is unique, there's a universal system to achieving terrific hair.

Finding a great stylist is always important, but you've got to have a stylist that can make your hair user-friendly. Your style won't be of any use to you unless you learn to manage it yourself. Find a stylist who will show you how to take care of your hair between visits. There are wonderful stylists out there. Some will even show you how to cut your own bangs, because they know you'll try to do it yourself anyway. Don't go longer than six to eight weeks between cuts, even if you're growing a style out.

Always use your fingertips, not your nails, to wash your hair. The water shouldn't be too hot, and you should add a tablespoon of apple cider vinegar to your final rinse for shine and to get rid of residue.

Massage your scalp while shampooing to encourage hair growth. Usually when men or women start to lose their hair, they're afraid to touch it, but that's the wrong approach. Massaging also gets rid of product residue lurking in the scalp that inhibits hair growth. It's also important to massage the scalp to increase circulation. The scalp is the only area of the body that doesn't have muscle directly beneath it.

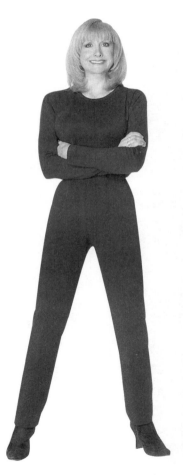

Diane's Tips:

SHOPPING SKILLS

To become a shopping master, you first need to shop your closet. That's right, you really don't know what you "need" until you see what you have! Never shop without a list, otherwise you're going to "impulse buy" useless items that you'll never wear. I teach my clients to keep an ongoing list by the closet door.

Your best bet is to shop stores with large inventories. Even their sales area will have a better selection than "off price" merchandisers who carry a little of this, and a lot of "that."

If you've discovered a designer that provides you with a great fit, then first shop that department. Not only will it speed things up, but the colors will probably coordinate, even season to season.

No matter how rushed you are, don't buy it unless you've tried it on.

Make sure you look fabulous from every angle.

Rely only on a three-way mirror.

The look has to be a total success, coming and going.

Sales are a mixed blessing. If you truly love something, don't wait and hope for it to go on sale. This is especially true of a great jacket, a basic skirt or pant, and comfortable, yet stylish, shoes. What you should really never pay full price for are basics like t-shirts and workout wear. When they do go on sale, stock up. You can also get them in bulk at mass merchandise stores.

Even though you've gone through these steps, before you buy, be sure that the store offers a full refund policy.

Don't take the tags off until you're sure you love it.

Hang it in the closet with similar colors, and try it on again with everything you wish to match up with the piece.

Unless it goes with at least two items, you really need to take it back. It won't be worth the cost per wearing.

My Journal:

Take a step back and look at your approach to each meal of the day. Look not just at what you eat, but at the times you eat and your eating environments. Write down how you felt after each meal. Are there any negative patterns you could break?

Breakfast:

Where? _____ What time? _____

Feelings after eating:

_____

Snack:

Where? _____ What time? _____

Feelings after eating:

_____

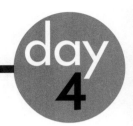

day
4

Lunch:

Where? _____ What time? _____

Feelings after eating:

_____

Dinner:

Where? _____ What time? _____

Feelings after eating:

_____

Makeup Basics

Applying makeup is not hard to do, as long as you have the right techniques to guide you.

☑ For great lashes combine mascara brands. Start out with one that separates lashes so they stand out. Follow with a coat of one that thickens, so they're full.

☐ Eyebrows look best when filled in with a soft pencil, then softened with powder.

☐ To get the best curl from your lash curler, use a blow-dryer to heat curler for about five seconds before using.

☐ Pull your eyelid taut when applying eyeliner.

☐ Keep your mouth open when applying eye makeup. It keeps you from blinking.

☐ Bend the tip of your mascara wand until it's angled to resemble a dentist's mirror. The wand will be easier to control, and the brush will provide better coverage.

☐ Apply yellow eye shadow on your lips as a primer to warm up lipstick color.

☐ Apply lip pencil in dots around your lips, then connect the dots following your natural lip line.

☐ Peach blush is universally the most flattering to skin, including women of color.

☐ Brush powder only on the center of your face. The sides of the face are always drier and don't require it.

day four
my diet today

Breakfast: _____
_____

Lunch: _____
_____

Dinner: _____
_____

Snack: _____
_____

Glasses of Water:
☐ ☐ ☐ ☐ ☐ ☐ ☐ ☐ ☐ ☐

Camouflage Camp

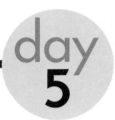

Before we start to camouflage your imperfections, we need to figure out if what you're so ashamed of is really a flaw. We're defining new ways of being beautiful, so what you might think of as unsightly, others might wear with pride. Just ask Madonna what she thinks about the gap between her teeth. Or ask Jennifer Lopez if she wants to make any excuses for her ample assets.

Freckles can look cute and natural, so why are you trying to hide them? A big smile reflects a warm, friendly persona. So smile away! You may be hiding your best assets because it's not fitting into some imagined standard.

Don't wait until you've lost any of the weight you intend to drop before you start dressing up and showing off. You can look ten, or even twenty, pounds thinner by mastering the art of camouflage. In doing so, you'll feel more attractive and be inspired and excited to stick with your goals.

Techniques and Tips

- You can draw up your eyes and give yourself a virtual face-lift with eyebrow camouflage alone. Simply arch your eyebrows with slanted tweezers, and fill and shape them with pencil. Soften your brow with matching eye shadow. A harsh brow looks unnatural and "mean." By bringing attention to your brow, you also take attention away from a double chin or puffy cheeks.
- You can appear to lose weight in just minutes. You'll be amazed at how just pulling up your bra straps will allow you to look taller and slimmer while giving you better posture.
- Don't wear anything too large or bulky in an attempt to camouflage excess weight. It makes you look even bigger! Remember this rule: if one piece of an outfit is roomy, then the other piece should be lean.
- Small shoulder pads can pick up drooping shoulders, but large shoulder pads should be avoided. Although they may appear to add balance, they're really only adding bulk.
- Show off skin in places you like, like a great neck or really good legs. Then cover what you're working on right now.
- Dark hose allow heavy legs to look long and slim, especially when matched to shoes.

PLAY UP YOUR STRENGTHS, PLAY DOWN YOUR FLAWS.

- V-necks and scoop necklines create a vertical line to camouflage chubby necks. Even lightweight knits can be slimming when they skim over the body rather than cling.
- Wear shoes with a chunky two-inch heel to make your legs look longer. Very narrow heels are only for very slim legs. Delicate shoes will make thick ankles appear even thicker, not to mention the danger of turning your foot in them.
- Dress in one color from head to toe to trick the eye. It's called monochromatic dressing. Wearing one color from shoulder to shoe streamlines the body, and is considered to be the ultimate thinning camouflage. If you want to take this look to the limit, choose dark, matte, matching colors.
- Camouflage for the workplace follows similar guidelines. Straight-cut, fingertip-length jackets cover everything up nicely. Coordinate it with flat front pants. Stay away from cuffs or any other detail that shortens the leg. Flat textures do the best slimming, and light wools create an elegant look.
- For large sizes (18 and up) don't fall into the trap of wearing oversized, tentlike clothing. Look for jackets designed with a subtle nip at the waist. Pants that have a slight drape and flow will be the most flattering style for you. Tops that stop right at the widest part of the hip should be avoided.
- Even the way you wear your hair can help to hide a double chin, wrinkles, aging, and weight. Your stylist should know how to begin layering right at the jawbone, just below the ear lobe, and finish layering below the chin. Full cheeks can become sculpted by creating angles from the temple to just below the cheekbones. Be aware that full, fussy hair looks outdated and unflattering. Go for sleek and managed styling.
- Hair coloring also has the ability to change the appearance of the face. Strategically placed highlights create long vertical lines and the illusion of slimness. Lightening your hair by a shade or two will open up your face and instantly slim down your cheekbones. Height at the crown of the head will dramatically lengthen your face.
- You can even give the appearance of longer, thinner hands with camouflaging techniques. Switch to a lighter shade of nail polish. Beige and neutral pinks will blend right into your skin. If your nails and hands are short, lengthen them by applying polish only on the center portion of the nail. Leave just a sliver of bare nail on either side.
- Create a temporary "pumped up" look. Just before you head out, hold a ten pound weight up and out to the side, bending your arm at the elbow. Slowly lower the weight. Repeat twenty times. Then, hold it behind your head with both hands. Slowly lower hands to the middle of the back. Be sure to hold your elbows close to your head. Repeat twenty times and you'll be looking so good!
- Fake long sleek legs by raising up on tiptoes for as long as you can. Try to go for a full minute. Go up and down quickly at least ten times. This will give your calves a firmer, more toned appearance.

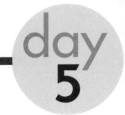

- If you want to achieve a more defined appearance of your buttocks, lie down with your legs raised in the air, knees slightly bent. Tuck your hands behind your head. Slowly lift your buttocks a few inches off the ground. Squeeze them together while you lift. Hold to a count of twenty. Lower slowly. Repeat twenty times.
- The right shoe can make your feet look an entire size smaller. T-strap sandals create a vertical line form ankle to toe. Strappy sandals, wedges, and platforms are slimming. Even a one-inch heel will make legs look leaner.
- Don't overlook the camouflage effects of undergarments. A mini control slip is short enough to wear under a short skirt, and it helps eliminate bulges from waist to thigh. A body shaper comes with convertible, removable straps to work with any dress style to create a long, smooth line. A body shaping slip is the ultimate body camouflage. Look for the style with a structured underwire bra built in. It shapes the entire torso to eliminate any bulges or bumps.

Camouflage from the Inside Out

While you're camouflaging your exterior features, it's time to work on what really matters, the inside.

If you're not feeling particularly attractive, then fake it. Soon, something will kick in, and you'll feel attractive. It's the concept of "fake it 'til you make it."

The concept has been around forever, and, rather than being "phony" or trite, I consider it to be survival in a world where the physical being is in competition with the emotional, intellectual, and spiritual parts of us. Wouldn't we love to go around with our spirit being our foremost image? But we live in a physical world, and appearances do count. In fact, they are the first and most lasting impression of any individual. Wear the joy and feel the perfection, and you might just trick your mind into being joyful and feeling perfectly wonderful for being you.

Around the home, you can also camouflage your surroundings with flowers, candles, and scents. It is amazing how these simple pleasures can lift your spirits. Remember, camouflage is only temporary while we fix things on the inside.

When in doubt, remember, the ultimate camouflage is a smile!

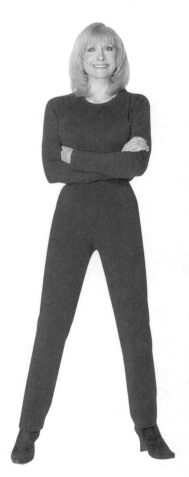

Diane's Tips:

GO FOR THE BRONZE

Makeup can dramatically slim down the face.
A makeup artist's best friend is bronzing powder.

For example, you can slim down a nose by running bronzing powder down the sides. Even if you've got chipmunk cheeks, you can create the illusion of cheekbones in a subtle and believable way by running the bronzer right under the cheekbone area. Feel around. Yes, they're really there. You'll locate them! Keep looking!

Disguise a double chin by running the bronzer all along the jaw line. Head to your local drugstore and pick up an inexpensive brand. It's not necessary to spend a lot since you're not really looking to get color or lots of pigment from your bronzer. You can also use face powder in a color that is one or two shades deeper than your foundation if you prefer a more subtle appearance.

PHOTO FINISH

Can you camouflage your body for a great picture?
Models do it all the time.

First, use lots of powder. Most cameras will make you look shiny. Apply concealer right under your brows to make your eyes appear bigger. Avoid dark lipstick if the film is black and white. Create darker brows. They tend to fade out in photos. Use shine or shimmer in only one or two areas. It reflects light and is exaggerated in photos.

To position yourself, place your hands on your hips so there's a space between your arms and your body. Drop your chin and stick your tongue on the back of the roof of your mouth. Models do this to give definition to their jaw lines.

Don't smile too broadly, it gives you the appearance of chipmunk cheeks. Smile as if there are weights on either side of your mouth. That's plenty of smile and it won't result in squinty eyes.

My Journal:

Look in the mirror and study your features. Pick out your three best features and list them in order of preference. These are the features you'll want to play up more prominently.

1. _____
2. _____
3. _____

Now pick out the three features of your face or body you consider least attractive. This will help you determine what you want to camouflage.

1. _____
2. _____
3. _____

Practice a camouflaging technique on your face. What did you try and how did it work? How will you do it differently next time?

_____
_____

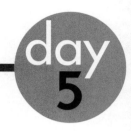

Try fixing a flaw of your body. Does your camouflage technique make a difference? Describe the difference.

_____
_____
_____
_____

Envision yourself in your dream outfit. What is it and what do you need to do to make it look great?

_____
_____
_____
_____
_____
_____

Boot Camp Basics:

Style Basics

Throughout Beauty Boot Camp, you should care intensely about your appearance. It is easier to lose weight when you look and feel attractive.

- ✔ Match your hose to your shoes. Legs look longer and thinner when hose is toned to skirts and shoes.

- ☐ Use a shirt like a jacket or tunic. Wear it over slim pants.

- ☐ Wear control top pantyhose with plenty of Lycra.

- ☐ The most flattering fabrics, such as light woolens and rayon, drape the body.

- ☐ Shorter length skirts and dresses make legs look longer.

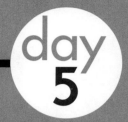

☐ Vertical buttons and seams lengthen the torso area.

☐ Simple styling is most slimming. Cuffs, pockets, and buttons add width to the body.

☐ Wear belts in a low slung manner, just below the waist.

☐ Wear opaque hose with short skirts.

☐ The more casual the look, the thicker the shoe heel. Always wear some kind of heel if
you can, even with pants.

day five

my diet today

Breakfast: _____
_____

Lunch: _____
_____

Dinner: _____
_____

Snack: _____
_____

Glasses of Water:

☐ ☐ ☐ ☐ ☐ ☐ ☐ ☐ ☐ ☐

Seize Control

TAKE

CONTROL

OF

YOUR LIFE

TO

DESTRESS

AND FIND

CONTENT-

MENT.

You can only gain complete control of your life and make the necessary changes by taking charge of everything that surrounds you. What you touch, what you feel, and even how you think contributes to your overall well-being. When you have a life that's disorganized and cluttered, it can drain your energy, and even make you sick.

What about your physical space? You most likely have enough of it, but you may be living in chaos. The simpler the space, the clearer your mind. It will be easier to make decisions and the right choices. A sloppy, cluttered environment spills over to other areas, causing stress and a lack of control, while a well-planned space eliminates stress and reduces negativity.

Small changes, such as putting a room together, can give you a sense of peace. For example, you should arrange seating around windows with the best views. Those windows should be cleaned and appointed with the least amount of window treatment possible. Letting in the light is good therapy, and it is especially important if you suffer from seasonal affective disorder.

Having beauty all around you will keep your mind on self-pampering and on track with your self-improvement mission. We admire art because of its great beauty. Not only do we want to become our own artwork, but everything around us should be feeding our spirit.

Kitchen Control

A totally clutter-free kitchen is one in which you can make clear choices about food. It should be both clutter- and stress-free. There should be no food in sight, except for what you're going to be eating in the next few moments. The exception to this rule is your next snack, for instance a piece of fruit you'll have between breakfast and lunch. If you have cookies on the counter, as well as an apple (your designated snack), guess where your eyes and your appetite will go.

I don't even recommend keeping decorative empty dishes or glasses around the kitchen. They subliminally beg to be filled. The exception, and a good way to keep your meals on track, is to set the table for your intended next meal. Use the very best place setting you can afford. You'll signal to your brain that your next meal is going to be breakfast the next morning, or dinner, not a bunch of junk in between. Even eating off nice china and sparkling silver and drinking from crystal glasses at a well set table will create peace of mind, which will cause you to eat more slowly.

- Keep non-food items in your kitchen for display. Flowers are aesthetically pleasing, and mirrors will bring new light into the kitchen.
- You should also have your kitchen stocked with your favorite free-for-all food items, so that when you do wander in, you can avail yourself of your favorite teas, chilled beverages, etc.

Your Destress Room

Create one room that has no clutter—a minimal amount of stuff—and use it for your escape. Sit in it, breathe deeply, feel that calm washing over you. Keep your journal in this room and take time in its calm to gather your thoughts before writing. If you can't spare an entire room, create a corner, or consider using the bathroom as your stress-free sanctuary.

- Here you'll connect with your inner wisdom, so the room should not have any distractions. There should be no TV or other noise. Use very soft and soothing music if you need it.
- You can use this space in the morning to strategize about your upcoming day or in the evening to review it. You may want to use the time to collect your thoughts, or just sit back and let your mind do the work for you.
- Some of us have a very hard time settling in. For us, there may be a need for a catalyst, such as a scrapbook of memories or old photos. This area would be a great place for wedding albums, yearbooks, and childhood tokens.
- You might want to fill this space with favorite scents or photos of places you would love to visit.
- Sometimes, you may wish to use your quiet time in this space to vent feelings, especially if something negative has been festering. A good cry can be cleansing. Just breathe, and let it happen.

Perhaps you would like to develop a daily ritual, like lighting a candle and imagining yourself with the strength and courage of a warrior. See yourself dancing through life, rather than sitting on the sidelines. You should sit back, close your eyes, and see the many ways you can use your abilities to make this world a better place. You'll feel connected to the world, which is especially important if you've been feeling isolated. Now, breathe out all the feelings of rejection and failure, and breathe in all the successes and opportunities waiting for you.

Personal Space

There are things in your personal space that you should have on hand for your convenience. You need to have these items out in the open or nearby in a container. Everything else should be in storage and clearly marked.

You've spent a small fortune on your things, so doesn't it make sense to keep them in excellent condition? The proper storage

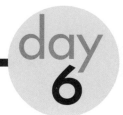

can make this possible. You take care of your car, your kids, and your friends. Why not give your personal space and its contents the same consideration? It doesn't take all that long, and it will make your life easier, because you'll be able to find what you have.

Getting your space together is even stylish! Choose storage containers that are decorative wherever possible. Baskets are an inexpensive way to store bathroom supplies and washcloths, as well as toiletries and magazines. If there is any item in your home that can hold things without breaking, it's a potential storage container. Be as creative as you are in your wardrobe!

Mind Control

To keep your mind free and focused, you need to give yourself the space to make mistakes. Allow yourself enough flexibility to be truly human. By forgiving yourself, you'll create an inner serenity and harmony that will become impenetrable. Set goals with those allowances.

If you tend to procrastinate, start with small, achievable goals, and then work your way up. I suggest you buy a timer and set it, leaving yourself no more than thirty minutes to do what you're reticent to accomplish. Once the time is up, you may find that you have the momentum to add another twenty minutes to your project. This is never truer than with exercise. No one wants to get started, but once you do, it's full steam ahead. It's all about setting your mind to it. If you can't do it right now, get that timer, and soon it will become habit.

Give yourself a deadline for something you've not been able to finish. If you find yourself becoming overwhelmed by a deadline, then break it down into smaller tasks. You have to have a game plan and specific goals. Write it down in outline form. Seeing it on paper will make it seem less scary.

You need to put your life in order. During Beauty Boot Camp we are doing lots of things, talking about many changes, but we have a specific mission—B.E.D. That is, beauty, exercise, and diet. Accomplishing these goals will be impossible without putting your mindset right on it. Getting on a treadmill when your mind is elsewhere just won't work.

If you truly want to change your looks, you need to visualize the changes. Every day, you should take the time to feel your feelings and set your mind to where you want to go. Do this in the morning, in the middle of the day, and just before bed. Train your mind to feel good about the unique person you are. Make your head store the positive thoughts and throw away the negative ones. Just try to tell a woman I've trained that she's not looking great—she'll check your glasses!

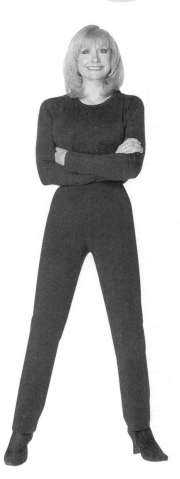

Diane's Tips:

PURSE CONTROL

Controlling your life away from home is all about your handbag.

You don't want to lug a purse full of things you don't need. It'll be heavy and cumbersome.

Purchase the lightest weight handbag you can find, while still getting the size you need. Pick it up and make sure it's not heavy before you fill it. There are some great bags out there, but what were those designers thinking? They're as heavy as suitcases! Instead, look for lines called "light weights" which are soft, light leathers that look even better the older they get. Microfibers are also wonderfully manageable.

Your handbag is the most important accessory in your wardrobe. It is near eye level, and is the first evidence of your taste. It's an old myth that you have to match your handbag to each and every outfit. However, there should be some coordination. Choose your bag in a neutral or multi-color shade so that it can go with the majority of your wardrobe.

Purchase the finest bag you can afford. You use it more than any other accessory, several times a day, so it needs to stand up to all the wear and tear. Find one with compartments, or put your items in separate compartments (pencil cases are great for this since they're transparent).

Here's what you'll need as a basic day bag:

a compact with a mirror and transparent powder • keys • breath mints • lipstick that can double as blush • a notebook and pen • a comb or brush • a wallet with space for credit cards and change • tissues • an address book

If you have room, include an eyeliner and neutral eye shadow that can double as lip powder. If you have lots of room, you may be able to throw in a sewing kit, mascara, and baby wipes for getting rid of stains and refreshing yourself.

The ultimate evening bag **should have some cash, lipstick, a compact, breath mints, and a comb.**

My Journal:

Today you created your special destressing place or room. Where is it?

_____

What did you put in your destress room and why? How do these things make you feel?

_____
_____
_____

Today you also began to focus yourself and give yourself the flexibility to find inner serenity. Answer the following questions to understand yourself better so you can avoid pitfalls and plan for success.

1. What tasks and activities do you eagerly do?

_____
_____
_____

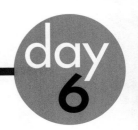

2. What tasks and activities do you procrastinate over?

_____

_____

_____

_____

_____

_____

_____

3. How can you positively reward yourself for doing the tasks you need to do, but about which you tend to procrastinate?

_____

_____

_____

_____

_____

_____

_____

Boot Camp Basics:

Diet Basics

These are tricks of the trade used by the world's best bodies.

✓
☑ Soy will do more for you than just help you have a fabulous figure. Soy is packed with powerful antioxidants that interfere with free radical damage.

☐ Scientists have discovered that a diet which contains chili, peppers, salsa, mustard, and ginger will provide a 45 percent increase in one's metabolic rate over a bland diet.

☐ Eat seed-containing fruits and vegetables, including the seeds themselves. Seeds are a great source of fiber and help foods to go through your body quickly.

☐ Candies and gums sweetened artificially can't be broken down in the body efficiently and can cause severe bloating.

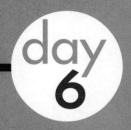

day
6

- Never eat anything bigger than your head, even lettuce. You'll only stretch your stomach out.
- Eat slowly. You'll enjoy your food more, eat less of it, and the extra chewing will relieve stress.
- Remember, your motto should be "diet one day at a time."
- Call a friend when you feel lonely. Food is not a companion.
- The way you breathe can give you energy that you thought could only come from food.
- Refrigerate your canned meats, soups, and gravies. The fat will collect and rise to the top so that you can scrape it off.

day six

my diet today

Breakfast: _____

_____

Lunch: _____

_____

Dinner: _____

_____

Snack: _____

_____

Glasses of Water:

☐ ☐ ☐ ☐ ☐ ☐ ☐ ☐ ☐ ☐

Reclaiming Self-Value

NURTURE

YOUR

PERSONAL

NEEDS

AND

PUT

YOURSELF

FIRST.

Self-value has nothing to do with how you look, it's about how you feel about yourself. It's about refusing to settle for anything but the best, because you are worthy.

Look around you. Who do you know that has a true sense of self-worth? They should quickly come to mind, because they're the ones who stand out. It's in the way they carry themselves, paying attention to the details most of us don't bother with or say we don't have time to take care of.

Let's talk about some celebrity women who appear to have so much self-worth, it's almost scary.

Madonna is not a natural beauty (self-admittedly), yet her looks are trend-setting and captivating. Madonna's a known risk-taker. She continually reinvents herself. She's fearless and adventuresome in her methods, to say the least. If you turn your head for too long, you may miss a look or two. You also may notice that she has embraced a couple of looks that just did not work for her. Did she come out worse for the wear? Of course not! She tries it, wears it for a while, fine tunes, and then goes on to something else.

Demi Moore has slowly evolved her looks. It's not so much that she's continually reinventing herself, but that she knows how to refine her looks.

Never let anything come between you and your self-worth. Don't allow anyone to make you feel less than you are. Schedule time with yourself and no matter what, show up! Ask yourself what makes you afraid to make a change and why.

Cultivating self-value leads to a wonderful sense of spiritual renewal. It frees you and brings you back to the time when you believed you were the center of the universe. Remember, it's only the externals of life that made you think differently.

Self Rituals

To start reclaiming your self-worth, it's necessary to get positive energy flowing throughout your body. Take off your shoes and stand with your feet shoulder-width apart. Bend your knees slightly and allow your hands to fall gently by your sides. Imagine you have a string coming from the top of your head. Pretend it's attached to the ceiling and is holding you upright. Relax your shoulders and neck. Stand and breathe naturally, being aware of each breath. Do this for about two minutes. Next, take deep breaths into the deepest part of your stomach (around the navel area). Keep breathing for another two minutes.

I first started using this technique when teaching posture to models. Many of them would report feeling an intense tingling going through their bodies. They would end the exercise feeling totally energized and self-assured. For the rest of Boot Camp (and beyond!) practice this technique each day. Not only will you have great posture, but you'll feel your self-worth emerge.

Practice positive reinforcement with your mirror. It may sound unbearable, but try standing naked in front of your mirror, and finding something new to like about yourself. Maybe it's your ears or your ankles. You have to like something you see there.

If you're totally stuck, draw a self-portrait with a plain piece of paper and a pencil or a crayon. Look at your picture. What appears normal and what is out of proportion?

Your drawing may be your subconscious speaking. The features you have drawn in the most normal manner are most likely the parts of you with which you're least concerned. These are the parts to flaunt. The ones that are oversized or disfigured are what you consider your worst features. These are the ones you need to work on or find ways to camouflage.

A Day of Self-Care

Can you really take care of yourself and get anything else done in your day? Yes, not only will putting yourself first allow you to get through your day, you'll get through it with more ease, and it will leave you with time left over to give to others.

The biggest obstacle to self-care during the day is change. The only certainty in life is change, and each day brings plenty of it. You just need to develop a plan so that these changes won't throw you off balance.

Whether you're at work, school, or home, you must maintain emotional balance to keep centered and stay whole. Your attention to self-maintenance will allow you to retain a position of power. You're most likely to leave Beauty Boot Camp when you're feeling tired and weak.

Of course you have to maintain a schedule, but you must leave time for life. You can still do a great job, but it will be consolidated into a certain time frame. Plan to work during your peak energy periods so that you actually give more to your obligations. Then rest, regroup, and evaluate when that energy drains.

Keep your body at its optimum performance level by making adequate time for meals and snacks. Take time to step back, breathe, and evaluate. You need to be sure that you're heading in the right direction and eliminating any obstacles to your progress. It may be helpful to have a list of things you need to get done for the day and to prioritize them. Check them off as you go. Seeing your accomplishments on paper will help you to focus.

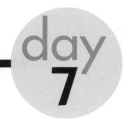

Don't take on more than you can handle. It's not the worst scenario if you have to push something over to tomorrow's list. Concentrate on your accomplishments and remember to treat yourself to some pampering, not only at night, but throughout the day.

Destress Yourself

There are things you can do to handle stress as it comes up rather than turning to food for solace. Loving yourself is so hard to do, and yet so necessary. Remember, nothing in your refrigerator ever loved you.

It's important to learn specific skills that will help you to reach your goals. If you use willpower alone, you're less likely to succeed. It's necessary to pull out every trick in your bag.

Although Beauty Boot Camp is only two weeks long, you're learning a lifetime of skills. This is not a one shot deal. You're learning to handle the means, so that the ends will take care of themselves. You need to get everything documented in your mind, and on paper. Focusing on your positive thoughts and attitudes towards yourself—and dealing with the negative ones—will heal you. Beauty alone will not make you happy. Think back to Marilyn Monroe, one of the greatest beauties of our time, and also one of the saddest. Looking your best only works when you're feeling your best.

Your knowledge of your body and its signals will help you handle your emotions and problems. When your stomach growls, you eat. When you're feeling a little upset, write it down, call a friend, or deal with it in your destressing place. If you need to change your location to get rid of the negative feelings, by all means do so. If you do find yourself drifting to food, ask yourself how eating is going to solve your problem.

Here's an exercise that is an alternative to nurturing yourself with food. Sit in a straight-backed chair. Take a deep breath and hold it for three to five seconds. Slowly exhale until you feel all the air leave your lungs. While seated, take another deep breath, and stretch your arms overhead, like you're trying to grasp something that's out of reach. Slowly exhale, and lower your arms. Now, bend over while you are still seated in that chair, reaching towards your toes. Sit back up, take a deep breath, and slowly exhale. Feel the calm wash over you, get up, and pass that fridge by.

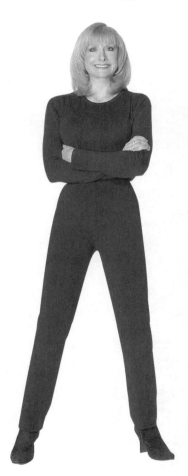

Diane's Tips:

SELF-CARE EATING

A diet never works when it's not made up of foods that you truly love.

It must also give you energy **and** vitality.

The foods you eat have the ability, directly and indirectly, to heal or harm you. Variety provides interest, enjoyment, and balanced, adequate nutrition. Eating under stress exhausts the body and shuts down the mind. It's no substitute for relaxation. Overeating is just one more pressure and stress that your body doesn't want or need.

Eating regularly and adequately is vital for energizing your mind and body. Meal times are an opportunity to slow down and rest. They are times to detach yourself from the day. They belong to you. Use them as positive reinforcement, and allow yourself to regroup.

In order to take care of yourself, it's important to enjoy this time. Appreciate each meal. Chew your food thoroughly to enjoy all its tastes and textures. The more attention, care, and time you give to eating, the better the food will be digested and do its work for your body.

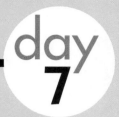

For starters, always use the best quality foods you can afford. You'll find yourself eating less because your satiety level will be reached more quickly.

Include fresh foods whenever possible. Many of the essential nutrients in foods are killed when they are cooked at high temperatures. Microwaving foods is another option. Fewer vitamins are destroyed by microwaving than by traditional cooking methods. Plus, many foods are actually more flavorful when they are microwaved.

You need to build your self-value in order to allow yourself to eat the right foods at the right tempo and to stop when it's the right time. You have to say to yourself over and over that you're truly worth it. And you can't just say it. You have to feel it, deep inside of you.

Practice until it becomes **real** to you.

My Journal:

List your three favorite things (make them tangible).

1. _____
2. _____
3. _____

If you can, keep these items nearby, especially in your destress place. Not all of our favorite things are tangible. Write down a favorite memory here.

_____
_____

Relate the following statements to something or someone.

_____ makes me feel good because _____

_____
_____

_____ makes me smile because _____

_____
_____

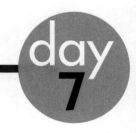

day
7

I feel/felt most attractive when:

_____

_____

I feel exhausted by:

_____

_____

I can overcome that exhausted feeling by:

_____

_____

I feel alone when:

_____

_____

Now, when I'm feeling alone, I will:

_____

Weighing In

Weight

———————

Waist

———————

Hips

———————

Bust

———————

Thighs

———————

Boot Camp Basics:

Energy Basics

You need to have energy to accomplish your goals. When you do, everything else is a little easier.

☑ Write out a schedule for your day and week, and prioritize what you need to do.

❑ Block out time frames for accomplishing tasks. Use a timer if necessary.

❑ Take a multivitamin to ensure proper nutrition.

❑ Wear comfortable clothing when exercising or working at your desk for long periods of time.

❑ Bring fresh air into your environment whenever possible. Open the windows, even for just a few minutes.

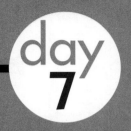

day
7

❑ Spritz your face with a water bottle for a quick refresher.

❑ When waiting in line, do calf raises. Stand up on your toes and hold for a count of ten.

❑ Always eat breakfast. It will keep your energy level up all day.

❑ Massage your scalp several times a day.

❑ Remember to stretch your body whenever you're talking on the phone or working at your desk for a long period of time.

day seven
my diet today

Breakfast: _____
_____

Lunch: _____
_____

Dinner: _____
_____

Snack: _____
_____

Glasses of Water:

☐ ☐ ☐ ☐ ☐ ☐ ☐ ☐ ☐ ☐

Survival Skills

Your total look is composed of many aspects. There is great power in every detail. Once you've honed the little details that help you perfect your total look, you'll feel unfinished without them. Your psyche will demand them.

In order to look and feel your absolute best today, it's necessary to have both a plan and a back-up plan—"survival skills," if you will. Wherever you go, be prepared with a survival strategy. Plan for trouble, and then take immediate action when trouble pops up. This rule applies to what you put in and on your body, on your face, and in your mind.

What does it take to survive in the world of beauty? Well, contrary to popular belief, it actually doesn't take a great face and a perfect body. What it does take is the power to optimize what you have. It's not necessary to apologize for wide hips when the beholder's eye is being drawn to those terrific legs.

Survival of the fittest is an individual matter. There are no set standards or stereotypes that you need to live up to. Your continued existence and growth in the world of physicality depends on your ability to project attractiveness no matter what you look like. It's this confidence that allows you to survive and feel comfortable in your own skin.

Femininity and sexuality transcend any clothing or cosmetic. I know I've been successful with a model when I can have her feeling so confident in her body that I can put even a garbage bag on her. She'll walk down the runway with her head up, shoulders back, stomach held in, rib cage raised, and make that bag look fabulous!

It's never been about what you wear, but how you wear it. And you know I'm not talking about your suits and jeans. I'm referring to your skin, your mind, your attitude, and your spirit. Yes, you can use tools to help your cause, but the greatest survival tool is YOU!

Hair Survival

Survival of the fittest hair states that less is more. Wash it less, brush it less, and put less stuff in it. Overambitious shampooing strips the hair of natural oils, making it dull and

PAY

ATTENTION

TO

THE

LITTLE

DETAILS

THAT

AFFECT

THE

TOTAL

PACKAGE.

71

porous. Not thoroughly rinsing out shampoo and conditioner creates build-up and residue and renders it unmanageable. Overzealous brushing causes unnecessary hair loss.

A poor diet directly affects hair, since hair is largely composed of vitamin B complex and protein. Choosing foods rich in these nutrients helps hair not only to survive, but also to flourish. Concentrate on foods rich in iron, like red meats. Add vegetables like carrots and broccoli. Fish should also be included. Check with your health care specialist about also including vitamin B and marine protein complex supplements.

When you do wear a hat, put your hair in a ponytail so when you take the hat off, you won't suffer from "hat head." Then bend over and flip your hair. Brush your hair from underneath to restore fullness.

The real survival secret is to recognize your hair type and use the tools and products that will keep your hair from letting you down. Follow the directions of the products you use on your hair. The ways in which the products are used, rather than the products themselves, usually make the difference in your results.

Exercise Survival

You know you need to exercise in order to get to the weight you want and then maintain it. It's a tool of survival for both your health and your looks. How much exercise is really necessary? The good news is that you may not need as much of it as you've been led to believe.

Whenever you move, you are exercising. You simply need to move in the most pleasurable and effective ways possible. It's the only way you'll be able to keep at it. Ignore the hype of the product pushers and personal trainers who urge you to spend an incredible amount of money on stuff you don't need and who design unrealistically time-consuming fitness routines. There's no way you could avoid becoming physically and mentally exhausted with what they suggest.

Not even celebrities and models could possibly keep up a three to four hour regime on a daily basis. Very few have the ability or the desire to spend that amount of time. When you do hear that they're going to such extremes, it's usually for an upcoming event.

Instead, do something you enjoy for thirty minutes a day. You can break it up into ten minute increments if you prefer, but it must be something you truly enjoy. It might be gardening or even active house cleaning. It might be mallwalking or taking the stairs instead of the elevator. Don't let your stair-stepper or your ab-roller become your lifeline. You need to rely on your determination and good sense.

You can carry your survival tools around with you, if it makes it easier. For example, keep a jump rope in your purse and get a few jumps in when you can. Wear ankle weights and work your legs when you're watching TV or talking on the phone. Keep weights in the kitchen or office, and while you're working, tone your arms.

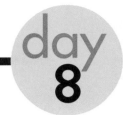

The time of day you exercise makes little or no difference in the quality of your results. What is most important is that you exercise when it's practical, and when you're most likely to do it.

Accelerating what you're already doing will help tremendously. Almost everybody walks somewhere. The easiest technique for increasing the fat burning effects of exercising is to turn up the voltage of whatever you normally do. Add hand weights and walk faster. You'll feel invigorated and pumped!

Diet Survival

Special problems arise that challenge even the most motivated dieter. A survival tool that you already own is the power of your voice. Bingeing can become so seductive and automatic that it sends the dieter into what I call a "binge reverie." When this happens, put your food down, stand up and yell "STOP!" You've awakened yourself from that semiconscious state that can lead to damage.

To help with chocolate cravings, use chocolate syrup in moderation. Another good substitute is diet hot chocolate. A chocolate Tootsie Pop has only sixty calories if you get stuck.

How do you survive airplane food? Plan ahead by requesting a special meal when you're making your reservations. It takes just seconds and saves an average of five hundred calories per meal. Most airlines offer both vegetarian and low-fat meals. You'll get an entrée that includes fruit instead of cake or a cookie. You'll also be served fresh vegetables instead of chips or crackers. Another benefit is that you're usually served first.

Cooking for a family can test even the most dedicated Boot Camper. You want to cook what they love, but you often end up tasting and testing the very foods you've been trying to avoid. Having something nearby to sip, like tea or bouillon, or chewing gum may help reduce your tendency to sample.

While making a meal, try to include at least two dishes that you can eat. Learn to cook more simply by broiling meats, cooking without a lot of oils, and serving sauces on the side. Add flavor with no-calorie zests and spices.

Even if you're on a tight budget, you can eat healthily and lose weight. Some of the most nutritious foods are also the least expensive. For example, beans, lentils, frozen fish, and tuna are tasty and economical. Avoid waste by cooking large portions and freezing the rest. Fruits and vegetables in season are usually cheaper than the packaged variety. If you have room to grow your own foods, you'll eat more healthfully, save money, and get exercise.

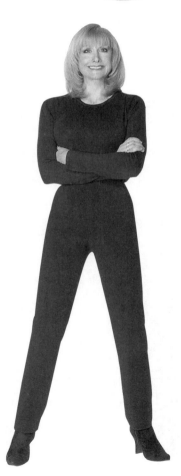

Diane's Tips:

DAILY SURVIVAL TIPS

There's no excuse not to look your best on a daily basis. Life is hectic, as we all know, but streamlining beauty and diet has never been easier. Keeping things simple makes survival less of a hassle and more of a treat. Don't worry about looking perfect, just jump in and do your best.

If you find yourself without a toothbrush, rinse your mouth with water and rub your teeth with a paper towel or tissue. It will help neutralize acids and reduce bacteria.

When there's no time to shampoo, mist your hair with water to bring back some of its natural texture. Comb through your hair with your fingers and then blow dry it or allow it to dry naturally. Spraying on a leave-in conditioner can help bring back some of your style's definition.

When there's no time to blow dry your hair, you can actually skip it all together if you style your hair with a wide-tooth comb while it's still wet. Comb a glossing gel through your hair, smoothing as you go. Your hair will dry totally styled.

Using one color is a time-saver with both your wardrobe and your makeup, and it looks more finished. A bronze lipstick can work as a shadow, blush, and a lip color. By sticking to one color scheme, a basic pant or skirt, matching hose, and shoes added to any top will look complete.

Survival on a daily basis works best when there's less to deal with. Simplify your beauty tools by using your fingers instead of a plethora of brushes and applicators.

My Journal:

Write down an emergency plan that will save you precious minutes and get you out the door in the morning quickly.

_____

_____

_____

Try it and time it: _____

What were the results? If they weren't perfect, were they passable? Would you save time by skipping or condensing the same things again?

_____

_____

_____

_____

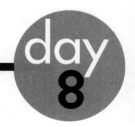
You may wish to have "survival packages" stashed in places you need them most, such as in your car, dorm, office, etc. List where you need them and what they will contain.

Area #1: _____

Supplies: _____

Area #2: _____

Supplies: _____

Area #3: _____

Supplies: _____

Today, at the midpoint of Beauty Boot Camp, double check that you are getting the right amount of water every day by looking back through your diet entries. Are you getting in eight to ten glasses? _____

Boot Camp Basics:

Finishing Basics

Show me a well-dressed woman, and I'll show you someone who has mastered the fine art of accessorizing. Accessories are the finishing touch that give us our individuality and show just how far we can go with a little imagination.

☑ Shoulder bags are most practical. Be sure the handles fit neatly over your shoulder and that the bag's bottom ends at a flattering height for your body.

❑ Use reinforced toes in your hose when not wearing open-toed shoes.

❑ Handwash hose in mild detergent.

❑ Don't wear dangling jewelry at work.

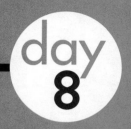

❑ One or two pins are a conversation starter. Several are a walking jewelry chest. The same rule applies to earrings, bracelets, and rings. Less is more.

❑ Feel free to mix real gems with simulated ones.

❑ Save large crystal jewelry solely for the evening.

❑ Coordinate your jewelry with your belt. Both are important accessories.

❑ Don't wear a daytime watch with evening attire.

❑ Use only skin-toned hose when wearing bright colors.

my diet today

Breakfast: _____

_____

Lunch: _____

_____

Dinner: _____

_____

Snack: _____

_____

Glasses of Water:

☐ ☐ ☐ ☐ ☐ ☐ ☐ ☐ ☐ ☐

Diane Irons' 14-Day Beauty Boot Camp

Daily Diligence

Every day you're getting better. You're developing your priorities and soaring to new levels. Remember: your top priority should be you.

Find out what you need to add to your routine or outlook that will get you to the next level, but don't fall into the trap of adding too much at once. A simple plan can carry you through each day and will be easier to manage. Cram too much into your regime, and you'll be less likely to maintain it.

Be flexible. Be spontaneous, and do something just a bit different every day to combat boredom.

Be diligent in checking for warning signs that you're really heading off track. It's a really big red flag when you see a pattern of lapses. Are you going out with unmanageable hair? Are you forgetting to floss at least once a day? Are you neglecting to drink your water? Fix it immediately. And then slow down so you can fit it in to your routine. Let go of whatever's keeping you from it.

Also, let go of a part of your routine that is unmanageable. It will become more trouble than it's worth. If it's something that can be done by someone else, then, by all means, seek support. It might be that no matter how hard you try, you just can't do a manicure on yourself that looks even vaguely presentable. Try enlisting a friend, or if that's not an option, have it done professionally. Do what you do well or can learn to do. Allow yourself the flexibility to succeed.

Diet Diligence

Each day you face the challenge of making the right choices in a world filled with many fat-ladened temptations. The good news is that you are not on the old standby diet that severely rations calories, making it harder, rather than easier, to lose the weight and keep it off. You will find that choosing the right foods will actually boost your body's ability to burn fat. Dieters who eat more low-fat foods lose weight more efficiently than those who select a diet that is lower in calories and higher in fat.

Have a plan to top your list with the foods that stimulate the body to lose weight. Grains are a must and should include cereals, oatmeal, popcorn, and corn. Don't miss out on the fruits that will satisfy and slim, including apples, cherries, oranges, grapefruit, and even the much maligned banana. Keep broccoli, spinach, carrots, and green beans as staples for your diet.

Snacking allowances must be made each day. Choosing snacks with negligible calorie counts will lead to burning almost as many calories chewing and digesting them as they actually contain. Keep these snacks in your fridge, on your counter, at work, and even in your car. Zucchini sticks are satisfying, easy to keep, and a cup will only set you back about eighteen calories. A cup of cucumber slices tastes great "as is," sprinkled with spices, or dipped in mustard or flavored vinegar.

The power of ice water cannot be overstated. Each day it will become so much a part of your regime that you'll start to feel thirsty without your eight to ten glasses. Remember, spicy foods will help you crank up your metabolism and keep your diet interesting.

Think about eating for beauty on a daily basis. Your diet can nourish your looks as well as your body. You'll become more beautiful as you slim down and stay at your optimal weight without feelings of deprivation.

Inner Diligence

I'd like for you to develop a mantra. Give yourself an empowering sentence or phrase that you can repeat under your breath when you are under stress or in times of success.

Write it down in your journal. It will help you when you are combating your inner demons that tell you you're not good enough, as well as those beauty bashers who enjoy bringing you down. Treat yourself with respect, and you are much less likely to let anyone else treat you badly.

At least twice a day, use your mantra to reinforce your dedication. Set aside five minutes to center yourself. Take this time to recheck your makeup, touch-up your hair, bring your shoulder blades back, and check your attire.

No matter how you started out your day, circumstances can bring both physical and mental changes. A touch-up is both warranted and beneficial. Taking time for your beauty routine provides you with the confidence to face the world as you never have. Confident women often experiment and primp as a way of boosting morale.

Style Diligence

Style is unique to the individual who has it. It would take forever to define it, and just as long to list its merits. I certainly can tell you what style does. It shines through your clothing and makeup. Each person should have a style they can call their very own. Although it's always important to stay up-to-date on trends, those trends should be adapted to fit into your own style. You'll know you've found a look that works well for you when you receive compliments on your "look" rather than your outfit du jour.

When you've found something that elicits compliments—it could be an outfit, a hairstyle, etc.—repeat it. Ask a friend to take pictures of you from different angles. See what you did differently, and then duplicate it. If it's a certain style of jeans, go grab a

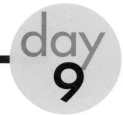

couple pairs. If it's a great hairstyle, bring that picture back to your stylist. She may not remember what she did before, never mind trying to duplicate it sight unseen.

How can you tell if you possess a timeless style or are just stuck in a beauty rut?

Some of us get our routines down pat, fall into that comfort level, and stay with those products and routines forever. If someone remarks that you "never change" as opposed to "you look so great," then try something new. Have something done professionally if you've been doing it yourself. Part your hair in a different way. If you've been known for a matte, sophisticated look, add some shine.

It's as important to be remembered for your style as it is for your wit. You may have developed and kept a look because of peer pressure, culture, or even family dictates. Search for the origins of your own style.

A playful style will boost your confidence and honor your uniqueness. Don't be afraid to make a mistake. Your looks can be changed as quickly as you change your mind.

Exercise Diligence

It's difficult to stay inspired day after day about improving your diet. It's even harder when it comes to exercise. The right friend can make all the difference in the success of a daily exercise regime.

If you have met anyone who has commiserated with you on their own weight struggles, that's a person to recruit. You may know somebody who doesn't particularly have a weight problem but loves to be competitive. They will inspire you as long as they don't sabotage you with their competitive spirit.

You may also want to recruit your entire neighborhood or office for a noon-time workout. All you need is a good pair of sneakers and comfortable clothing. If you can't get out of your home because of time constraints or small children, learn to improvise. Take a bath towel and lie with it lengthwise under you. Holding each upper corner of your towel, do sit ups and work your abs. The towel will support your head. While you're in your kitchen, use soup cans, soda bottles, and even milk cartons as improvised weights. A sturdy kitchen step stool can be used to strengthen your buttocks and thighs.

Cleaning is also a great workout. Do your squats while you're doing your laundry. Get a great workout in your garden by pulling weeds and working your arms. Raking will work your stomach and strengthen your back.

Just think about all you do and incorporate exercise into your day. You won't even need to change your schedule!

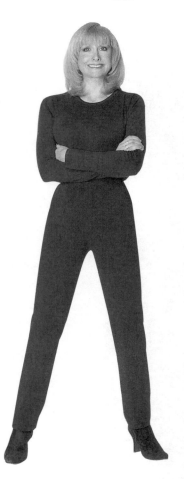

SKIN DILIGENCE

Each day, it's necessary to keep your skin protected from the effects of the environment with a regime that **corrects as it conceals**. There's no room in your skin's health for excess sunbathing, going to sleep without properly cleansing, or worse, attempting to manually extract pimples and blackheads.

Skin properties change on almost a daily basis. Your skin care regime needs to be equally adaptable. It should vary according to the weather, your menstrual cycle, your mood, your diet, and on and on. You name what's going on in your life, and it will somehow affect your skin.

You should remember to use **sunscreen** with a **minimum SPF of 15**. It may be easier to find a sunscreen with moisturizers than a moisturizer with this much sun protection. Your local drugstore has several brands to choose from.

Your cleansing regime exists only to remove surface debris and oils, nothing more. This rule goes for the face only, but there are also cleansing rules for the entire body.

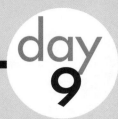
Water in the tub or shower needs to be comfortable and warm, but never hot. Extremely hot water can drain energy, rather than restore it. Plus, it dries out the skin.

The **type of soap** you use on your body varies as to where on the body you're using it. You actually need two different soaps in your bath. A deodorizing soap should be used only on the parts of your body that create odors. This soap would be used in intimate areas, feet, under arms, and under the breast area. A milder soap should be used on your legs, arms, back, etc.

Your skin is a direct reflection of your life.

Treat it with tender loving care and you'll put your best face forward.

My Journal:

Write down your mantra:

_____

_____

_____

Why did you choose this as a mantra? How does it make you feel?

_____

_____

_____

Now create a war cry that will stop you from doing something that will break your program. Be sure to use strong words in your war cry, such as "Stop it!" "No!" or "Never again!"

_____

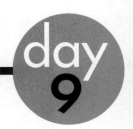

What are the looks on which you receive compliments? They can be specific outfits and accessories, or a more general style.

_____

_____

What can you do to incorporate more of those elements or looks into your style?

_____

_____

What tasks, trips, or chores do you do often that could be accelerated or augmented to make them more exercise-oriented?

_____

_____

Anti-Aging Basics

It is possible to extend our youthful looks with proper care and techniques.

☑ Avoid the sun and wear sunscreen. Exposure to the sun is the number one reason skin ages.

☐ Smoking causes early wrinkling by reducing the level of oxygen in your body. Drink lots of water if you're in the process of quitting.

☐ Alcohol in excess dehydrates the body and robs it of vitamins that keep skin both healthy and glowing. Follow each alcoholic drink with a glass of ice water.

☐ Purchase a magnifying mirror to see things happening to your face that the aging eye can't see.

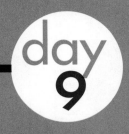

☐ Update your makeup the way you update your wardrobe.

☐ Don't stop changing or you'll end up a caricature of what you were at twenty or thirty.

☐ Regular exercise and meditation will help diffuse the effects of stress, which ages the body and face.

☐ Keep your chin from sagging by trying to touch your nose with your tongue whenever you can think to do it. Try to work up to fifty repetitions a day.

☐ Make dinner the smallest meal of your day. Your aging body needs extra time for digestion.

day nine
my diet today

Breakfast: _____

_____

Lunch: _____

_____

Dinner: _____

_____

Snack: _____

_____

Glasses of Water:

☐ ☐ ☐ ☐ ☐ ☐ ☐ ☐ ☐ ☐

Self-Defense

Today we're going to plan defense strategies, because no matter what we do to look and feel as good as we can, life happens.

You must take it easy in this program, or you'll surely run out of fuel. Beauty Boot Camp is fast and furious, but as with anything, cut yourself a little break now and then or you'll fizzle out.

One lapse won't hurt a two-week program, but the fewer slip-ups you have, the more likely you are to feel good about yourself and forge on. When you feel on the verge of overeating, keep your hands busy by doing your nails. Maybe your stress level is over the top. Calm your nerves by catching a movie or renting one. Do you need to take your mind off food? Send your appetite in another direction by absorbing yourself in a steamy love story.

You may find it more helpful to schedule your daily indulgences. It will give you something extra in the day to look forward to.

Remember, self-indulgence is not the same as sabotaging yourself. Get to know the difference, and you'll keep yourself healthy, beautiful, and guilt-free!

Prevention

A little planning will help prevent minor beauty issues from becoming recurring annoyances or things that get in the way of your total look.

For starters, if you've been ill and still must face the world, plan to bring some preventive measures with you. Carry a metal spoon and run it under cold water or keep it in a glass of ice water. Hold it wherever your face is puffy. Refresh your face throughout the day by carrying a spritzer bottle filled with cooled chamomile tea. The chamomile will calm down the puffiness and redness, while the water will keep your skin hydrated.

If your lips have a tendency to bleed, use concealer all around your mouth. Then apply a soft lip liner all over the lip, and finish with a touch of gloss to spread. You can apply lipstick, even without a mirror, by carefully dabbing lipstick along the bottom lip and on the bow of your upper lip. Rub your lips together to blend.

You can even defend against the loss of your fragrance by layering it. Begin with a shower or bath gel in your favorite scent. Use the same scent and apply your body lotion.

DEFEND

YOURSELF

AGAINST

UNEXPECTED

CHALLENGES

AND

SELF-

SABOTAGE.

Your skin should be slightly damp to help it absorb. Apply the scent itself wherever skin is warmest. Use it behind your ears, on your wrists, your décolletage, and behind your knees. The heat generated in these areas will keep fragrances on much longer.

If your skin tends to be dry, dab a bit of petroleum jelly to the pulse points of your body. This gives the scent something to which it can adhere.

Menu Attack Strategy

To successfully maintain a healthy, balanced diet every day, you must map out your menu. When you can plan your meals ahead of time, you don't have to deal with how many grams of protein are in this meal, or if you got enough calcium. It's been done for you in Beauty Boot Camp. Quite frankly, the less you need to deal with as you revamp and reevaluate your life, the easier and more organized everything will seem.

But when we're done, you need to prepare a healthy balanced diet for yourself. To defend yourself against failure, you must plan it out. If you're proactive with your planning, you won't be reactive in your eating.

Food Defense

Who would dream that you'd ever have to defend yourself against food? It's not food in general, but specific techniques that allow for self-defense dieting. For instance, there are some special items you will need to purchase in order to make the right choices meal after meal. Make sure that they're at the top of your shopping list.

Enjoy a variety of both cold and hot foods. The combination of both will be more satisfying. Your bread also will be more satisfying if you put it into the microwave for a few seconds. Plus, you'll enjoy the taste of the bread itself, and not need butter or other fattening spreads.

The fat content in meat varies from one percent for four ounces of skinless turkey breast to a whopping nine percent for four ounces of beef sirloin. You should be able to check it on the meat's packaging.

Don't bog yourself down with stuff that doesn't matter. For example, although it's absolutely important to eliminate fat in our diets, don't worry about putting whole milk in your coffee. You only save about four calories per cup. So if you feel that your coffee is too watery without that whole milk, pour a little in, and leave out the guilt.

Look for color when it comes to putting together a salad. The darker the color, the higher the vitamin and mineral content. Romaine and loose leaf lettuce have a much better nutrient value than the typical iceberg lettuce.

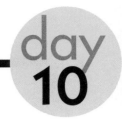

You can even enjoy dessert if you feel it finishes a meal. A little Cool Whip on top of sugar-free Jello sets you back only eight calories and tastes decadent! A little orange marmalade with orange liqueur over orange slices is one dessert even my "I've got a big photo shoot tomorrow" guests never refuse. Other fashionable desserts include baked slices of apple with cinnamon and popcorn coated with cinnamon.

Defense Shopping

You need to protect yourself whenever you shop. As a consumer, you are often protected if an item you bought goes on sale within seven days from the time of purchase. Always save your sales receipts, and watch your newspapers for at least a week. Keep your tags around, and don't hesitate to bring the item back for the savings difference.

Most drugstores now have liberal return policies when it comes to cosmetics, so you can feel comfortable purchasing from them without trying out the color.

Take it home, and if it isn't what it looked like on the package, bring it back. Most drugstores that have this policy simply request that you keep the receipt and bring it with you.

Shopping for shoes is something that most women have no problem accomplishing. Unfortunately, many of us are purchasing the wrong size shoes. It's important to shop for shoes late in the day when your feet are swollen and at their largest. Never purchase a shoe that bulges over the welt of the shoe. If a shoe has to be broken in, pass it up. You really don't know how well it will break in. Check for quality by placing each shoe on the floor to make sure they sit flat. Hold the backs of the shoes together to check that they are of equal height.

When shopping for sandals, avoid tight or flimsy straps, and don't purchase sandals that cut into your bunions or callouses. If you can pull the insole away from the sandal, it means the manufacturer may not have used the right adhesive.

When shopping for a fragrance, be sure to try it out for at least thirty minutes. If a company doesn't offer you a sample to take home, then apply the tester to your wrist, neck, or crook of your elbow. If you don't have the time to wait, rub your hands together to create perspiration, and then add a few drops to your palm.

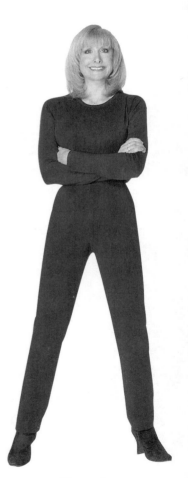

Diane's Tips:

HEALTH DEFENSE

Beauty without total health is incomplete. Defensive tactics must be followed in order to guard both your beauty and your health.

While I don't want you to feel as though you need to wear gloves and a mask in public, you can **avoid beauty-killing bacteria** by following a few fastidious rules.

For example, public restrooms are places where you can and should use extra care. They contain a lot of harmful bacteria. One rule is that it's safest to use the first stall since it's the one least often occupied, and least likely to be contaminated. After washing your hands, turn off the faucet with a paper towel.

Contrary to belief, **air blowers are not more sanitary than paper towels**. Blowers collect bacteria from the air and deposit them on your hands. Also, if you have to set your purse on the floor, place it on a paper towel. And don't touch the sanitary napkin disposal unit. Typically, it's not cleaned as often as the rest of the bathroom and is the most contaminated area in the entire restroom.

When you feel a cold or a virus coming on, act immediately. Sometimes, common household products are among the best medicines. For example, if you get a cold sore, place a dampened aspirin on it for about three minutes. Then cover it with some Pepto Bismol. Since it works on the virus of diarrhea, it can combat the cold sore virus.

When you feel a urinary tract infection coming on, call your doctor, and then grab some cranberry juice to start treating it.

Being proactive about your health
will contribute to glowing beauty both inside and out.

My Journal:

List a few things that could go wrong today.

_____

_____

_____

Now develop defense strategies for dealing with each of these things, either to prevent them or to handle them if they occur.

_____

_____

_____

_____

_____

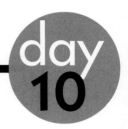

What foods do you enjoy that don't have a significantly negative impact on your diet and health goals? These are foods you can feel guilt-free about eating.

_____

_____

_____

What shopping mistakes have you made in the past? Did you buy wrong sizes or styles, or was there something else that was wrong with it? What would you do differently if you purchased the same item again?

_____

_____

_____

Emergencies

How do you solve the unforeseen beauty crisis? You handle it right away. You use the most inventive techniques and whatever products work.

- ☑ Hide a pimple fast by applying an ice cube directly to the blemish for thirty seconds to take down the swelling. Follow with an eye redness reliever to take away the redness.
- ☐ No time to wash your hair? No problem. Clean it fast by wrapping the leg of an old, clean pair of pantyhose (it will absorb oils) misted with perfume (which breaks down oils while leaving hair with scent) around a brush and brushing from roots to ends.
- ☐ To treat chapped lips, mix baking soda with water to make a paste, massage it over your lips and wipe them clean with a damp washcloth.
- ☐ Perk up tired eyes by applying a dab of highlighting blush beneath your brow bone and blending. It works by attracting light toward your eyes.

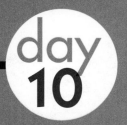
☐ Unstick a stubborn zipper by rubbing pencil lead over it, allowing an easy, smooth glide.

☐ Remove necklace knots by laying the chain on wax paper, placing a drop of olive oil onto the knot, and untangling it with two needles.

☐ Expand the waistline of a too-snug pair of pants or a skirt by slipping a rubber band through the buttonhole and looping it around the button.

☐ Handle a major breakout emergency by rubbing half a potato all over your face. Leave the raw potato juice on for twenty to thirty minutes. Rinse with cold water.

☐ Mix baking soda and hydrogen peroxide for use as an emergency teeth whitener. Be sure to keep this solution away from the gum area.

day ten
my diet today

Breakfast: _____
_____

Lunch: _____
_____

Dinner: _____
_____

Snack: _____
_____

Glasses of Water:

☐ ☐ ☐ ☐ ☐ ☐ ☐ ☐ ☐ ☐

Chemical Warfare

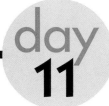

GET

NATURAL

AND

GET

REAL

ABOUT

BEAUTY.

Do your research and you'll often find that the core ingredients in a product are the ones that give it power. I've been on a personal crusade for quite a while to get my clients to take an extra minute or two and switch to natural ingredients. Your skin is not meant to have so many chemicals on it. Chemicals don't do much that's positive for your skin or body. Their purpose is often to give the product a shelf life. That doesn't help your skin.

The more you know, the more money you'll save, and the better you'll look. You'll feel like you're living at a spa. After all, at a spa you're always given the most natural treatments. Your ultimate beauty counter is your local grocery store. There you'll find fresh, natural treatments that will leave you refreshed and beautiful, both inside and out.

You'd be surprised at who uses grocery store beauty when they could easily afford the pricey alternatives. For generations, legendary beauties have carried their secret potions and treatments with them. They know these "special" treatments work better than many commercially available products and won't cause a bad reaction, which is especially important to those who make their fame and fortune from their fabulous faces.

On the other hand, I've had the loveliest models come to me with the scariest faces. They have either combined products that should not have been put together, or they're using a product that is just too strong for their skin type.

Making your own beauty products is not difficult. You can also add ingredients to basic products to create the same sort of effects that would cost you three times as much if you bought the product with the added elements. I'm referring to such things as vitamins. You'll see vitamins A, C, and E as additives in moisturizers. Unfortunately, these vitamins lose much of their potency when they are added ahead of time. They cannot remain stable even with the chemicals. Your best bet is to head to your favorite drugstore or vitamin shop and get capsules in the strongest formulation that you can find.

For instance, if you want to accelerate the moistening and healing effects of your moisturizer, simply put about a thimble full in the palm of your hand, empty the contents of a 1,000 mg capsule of vitamin E into it, and you'll feel the extra moisturizing right away! The same concept and technique applies to vitamins C and A.

Vitamins do a lot for your skin. Vitamin C is essential to the formation of collagen, which cements the skin cells together. It also shrinks pores by helping oil-secreting glands to properly function, protects the skin from sun damage, and fades age spots. Vitamin A regulates skin hydration and stimulates the growth of skin cells, as well as treating acne.

So start supplementing and saving your money and your skin!

Beauty from Nature

There are so many great products waiting for you at the grocery store. Start in the produce section and pick up some lemons. Use them to lighten various skin discolorations, or mix the juice with a little water to remove soap residue and grime. Add the juice to your shampoo for extra highlights.

If you have oily skin, grab an overripe tomato and remove the skin. Using a cotton ball, apply the tomato to a clean face. Leave it on for fifteen minutes, and then rinse with warm water. Tomatoes contain oil-absorbing acids and natural exfoliates.

Even potatoes are beauty enhancers. Raw potato slices contain potassium that effectively treats dark circles under your eyes. Lay down and place a potato slice under each eye, allowing the juices to be absorbed into the affected area. Tea bags also work because of their tannic acid components. Wet the tea bag and place them under your eyes, making sure they're cool to the touch.

Head to the dairy department and pick up some yogurt. When picking out your yogurt go for the added fat if you're only using it as a beauty treatment. Apply it all over your face to remove the dead cells and let it set for ten minutes. Use your hands and gently wash it off. The same applies to powdered milk, which is an excellent lactic acid wash and exfoliant.

Don't miss the cooking aisle. You'll find olive oil for damaged cuticles and dry skin. Solid vegetable shortening is fabulous as an intense moisturizer for hands, legs, and feet. Be sure to pick up some vanilla extract and use it in your bath as rich aromatherapy.

You'll love all the ways you can use natural products to treat acne. Take a little garlic oil and put it on an emerging pimple. Dab a bit of honey on a pimple and let it sit for ten minutes. Honey will deep-clean the pore and draw out bacteria.

Salt is also an effective beauty product. Soak a cotton ball in warm salt water. Press it on a pimple to dissolve the top. Add salt to your bath water, and it will stay nice and warm much longer.

Experiment with fruits of all kinds. For example, you can bleach out dark elbows by sticking each one in half a grapefruit. Sit and relax for about ten minutes, then rinse thoroughly.

Natural Teeth Whitening

It's easier than ever to have pearly white teeth, fresh breath, and healthy gums—and you can do it naturally!

Strawberries have gentle cleansing and bleaching properties and make a great natural teeth cleanser. Just crush the strawberries with a fork, and brush the pulp directly on the teeth. Rinse thoroughly. This delicious tasting "toothpaste" also helps remove coffee and tea stains that have formed.

Don't overlook the effect that certain foods have on natural teeth whitening. Foods such as spinach, lettuce, and broccoli prevent

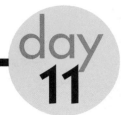
staining by creating a film on the teeth that acts as a barrier. There are some foods that work on the teeth like detergents. Foods that require a lot of chewing, such as apples, celery, and carrots, whiten teeth naturally.

You can even create natural mouthwashes. My favorite is the clove rinse. Simply heat a teaspoon of cloves with a half of a cup of water. It takes me about twenty seconds in the microwave, and then it cools down as I head to the bathroom. Let it cool completely and rinse your mouth thoroughly with it.

Another favorite of models is boiling a strong cup of peppermint or spearmint tea. Drink it in a slow and deliberate manner while rolling the tea around in your mouth.

You can also let the tea cool and use it as a regular rinse.

Natural Dieting

There are many foods that have direct beauty benefits working from the inside out. Carrots maintain the outer layer of the skin, and thus prevent premature aging. What is found in carrots is the similar to what you can get from Retin A.

Citrus fruits hold the skin cells together by forming collagen. Collagen cannot be added to the skin topically, which is why fruits and fruit juices are such an important part of your daily diet.

Sweet potatoes are an absolute must for many models. Christie Brinkley even cooks several at a time, and keeps them in her refrigerator for when she gets a sweet craving. You can also cook them ahead and quickly microwave them with a bit of cinnamon when your urge to eat something sweet comes up. Sweet potatoes are full of vitamin A, which is known to be a remarkable antiwrinkling agent.

Add leafy green vegetables and fresh fruits like peaches and apricots to your diet. These foods help prevent aging and repair the outer layer of the skin.

If you suffer from sallow skin, add a bit of lemon to your diet. Spritz it on your salads, add it to each glass of water, and flavor up your fish and vegetables.

Celery is a dieter's dream! Because it takes up so much space in your stomach, celery is one of the choice foods of the world's most beautiful bodies. It's a great source of fiber and a natural cure for constipation. It also contains both calcium and magnesium.

Try some unusual foods for variety. Figs are rich in niacin and magnesium. Experiment with mushrooms. They're great by themselves and can be added to antipasto and other vegetables.

Parsley has almost no calories and gives you the best breath! It's rich in chlorophyll.

Nutmeg is a natural sweetener and sunflower seeds are a great source of phosphorous. These are great foods that will directly contribute to even better looks.

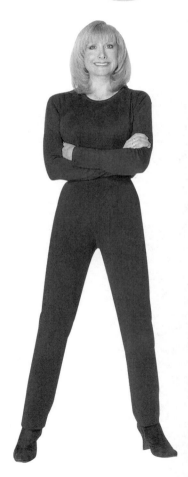

Diane's Tips:

NATURAL CELLULITE
SOLUTIONS

If you have cellulite, welcome to the club. Over 80 percent of women have this lumpy, bumpy skin. I've seen it on women of all sizes and shapes. What's the good news on such a nasty subject? There are natural and effective ways to diminish its appearance.

Caffeine is the first ingredient in most cellulite treatments. The same way caffeine gets us moving in the morning, it can also help to get our fat cells moving. So head to your coffee makers, girls, and go for the high octane stuff.

Do what famous models do ritualistically, and what beauty contestants do before that big swimsuit walk. Line your bathroom floor with newspapers, and then sit on the edge of your bathtub with used coffee grounds. Make sure that the coffee grounds are still warm, but comfortable, to the touch. If they've cooled down, simply heat them briefly in the microwave.

Rub them into the cellulite-laden areas of your legs using your hands or a loofah mitt. Although the grounds will pretty much hit the newspaper quickly, a residue will remain. Ideally, seaweed should be wrapped around the area to detoxify. If you are unable to find lengths of seaweed at your health food store or natural supermarket, use plastic wrap. Wrap completely around the upper leg and let set for a few minutes.

To intensify the treatment, take an old-fashioned rolling pin and roll the area to further smooth out the cellulite. Unwrap, brush the remaining grounds onto the newspaper, and rinse thoroughly.

For top results, you should do this treatment at least twice a week.

My Journal:

What chemicals have you discovered that you can eliminate from your diet?

_____

_____

_____

What products would you like to examine more closely to see if they are high in chemicals or more natural? Use creating this list as an action step to investigate these items.

_____

_____

_____

For which of your beauty care products could you substitute more natural alternatives? What is holding you back from switching to the natural alternatives?

_____

_____

_____

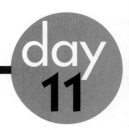
What "home remedies" have you or your girlfriends tried and found work better than store-bought products?

_____
_____
_____
_____
_____
_____
_____

Which of the natural alternatives mentioned in this chapter did you try? What were the results?

_____
_____
_____
_____
_____

Natural Basics

These kitchen cures can be even more effective than store-bought products at making your skin, hair, and nails look absolutely perfect.

✓ Get satiny skin with super moisturizing olive or vegetable oil and salt or sugar. Mix a half of a cup oil with enough salt (for dry skin) or sugar (for oily skin) to make a paste. Add a few drops of vanilla extract to leave your skin sweetly scented. Massage over your body while showering to remove flakes.

☐ Polish your skin with yogurt. It's loaded with exfoliating lactic acid. Plain yogurt sloughs away dry patches, while boosting moisture, and leaves your face with a healthy glow. Smooth one tablespoon yogurt over clean, dry skin. Let set fifteen minutes, then rinse.

☐ Eliminate ragged cuticles with a lime. It is chock full of citric acid, smoothing frayed cuticles instantly. It also brightens discolored nails.

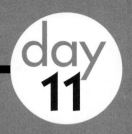

❑ Make blemishes disappear with toothpaste. It contains calcium carbonate, sodium bicarbonate, and carageenan (drying and purifying agents found in common acne treatments). Dab onto clean, dry skin. Leave on overnight with a bandage covering it.

❑ Fight dandruff flakes with mouthwash. It's the fast way to conquer dandruff because it's infused with an antiseptic that kills the dandruff-causing bacteria. Mix one part mouthwash with eight parts of water. Massage over clean hair. Wait five minutes, then rinse.

❑ Mash one scoop of ripe papaya with a half of a cup cornmeal. Replace in scooped out papaya and place elbows inside for ten minutes. Then brush mixture in with an old toothbrush. Papaya's natural enzymes will loosen the dead skin cells, and the cornmeal will slough them off.

❑ Black tea is high in tannic acid, which boosts the skin's moisture level. Saturate a black tea bag with very warm water. Press over clean lips for five minutes.

day eleven
my diet today

Breakfast: _____

_____

Lunch: _____

_____

Dinner: _____

_____

Snack: _____

_____

Glasses of Water:

☐ ☐ ☐ ☐ ☐ ☐ ☐ ☐ ☐ ☐

Budget Boot Camp

ADOPT

SUPER

STRATEGIES

FOR

SAVING

TIME

AND

MONEY.

Shake that dollar until it hollers! It's not necessary to spend a lot to look like you have. There's no reason you can't combine beauty with a tight budget. It may take a bit more time, but it's amazing how much you can save. Learn to read labels, cut out a few extras, and you'll be taking charge of your money.

Don't believe the hype. There's never been a direct correlation between the amount of money spent on an item and the degree of customer satisfaction. Educate yourself by taking notes about everything you see whenever you go shopping or have a service done for you.

Make notes at the hairdresser. See what products she is using and then find them for less at beauty supply shops. When you visit a cosmetic counter and see how the salesperson has done her eyes or lips, ask how she did it. Of course, she will show you with her particular line of products, but it's the technique that you'll copy. Then, go home and practice on your own face, using your own products.

Budget Wardrobe

If you're not particularly creative when it comes to wardrobe coordination, check how mannequins are dressed. Stylists are trained to dress them, and a salesperson can gather the look for you so that you can try it on in its entirety. Before you make the purchase, go home and see if you have some of the coordinating pieces at home. I like to take a digital camera with me to capture the look, and then bring it up on my computer. A simple Polaroid is a low-tech alternative

As you build your wardrobe, record your purchases so you don't end up duplicating anything. Keep track of your failures so you don't repeat your mistakes. Write down why it was a mistake. Was it the wrong color? Was it too small or too big? Did the trend go by too quickly to get your money's worth?

Or was the fabric all wrong? My idea of a fabric that not only doesn't flatter anyone but doesn't sound too attractive either is "wide wale corduroy." Remember, the fabrics you select can visually slim you down or bulk you up. It's not a bargain, no matter who the designer is, if the fabric doesn't flatter you.

You can assemble great basics with the right fabrics. It makes no difference if it fits perfectly or is put together exquisitely, it's the fabric that will make it work and bring you the biggest bang for your buck.

Budget Makeup

Endless possibilities exist for stretching your cosmetics budget. Makeup artists are known for creating custom colors on the spot, and it's a dollar-saving technique as well.

That color you are admiring on the cover of the latest magazine? It is very likely not available as a particular color in any store. It was designed for the model by a makeup artist from his or her own kit. And it's even more likely that the color that most flatters you is waiting to be created among the palate of colors you already have in your own makeup bin.

Remember, a little goes a long way when it comes to cosmetics. We waste so much as consumers, but cosmetics have to top the list. If you're like most people, there are one or two uses left in every one of your products when you throw them away. Over the course of a lifetime, you can save a lot of money if you learn how to reduce this waste and use products more efficiently. For instance, adding just a bit of water to your shampoos and conditioners can usually provide another application.

When makeup dries out before its time, don't throw it away. You can add a drop of water to your mascara wand, stick it back into the tube, and loosen the mascara that has dried out. You can stretch your foundation—and provide a more natural appearance—by mixing it with a little moisturizer. Do it in the palm of your hand, not the bottle. Spraying a fine mist of hairspray onto a powder puff will make the powder adhere to the puff so that it doesn't end up all over your clothing.

You can invigorate your manicure with shine serum. It works just as well on your nails as it does on your hair. It leaves your nails as shiny as when they were newly polished.

The best nail hardener available is also the least expensive. It's hoof lacquer, and you can purchase it at any drugstore. It was originally created to protect the hoofs of show horses. It will make your manicure or pedicure last twice as long. It's a big secret of top manicurists.

There are all kinds of samples that will allow you to try products without risk. Quite frankly, if it is possible, you should always try products before purchasing them. Simply look through your favorite fashion magazines and see what's being advertised. Tear out the pages and bring them to the cosmetics counter of your favorite department store.

Manufacturers generally stock these counters with their latest products so that salespeople will give them out to their customers. When you're making a purchase, they'll throw in these samples. If you're not making a purchase, you're going to have to ask, but the salespeople are usually happy to comply with your request. I love these samples as travel sizes in my purse and luggage. Many manufacturers now have Internet sites where you can sign up for samples, too. Often, you'll receive them by mail before they're even offered for sale.

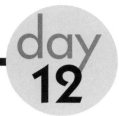

Budget Dieting

It's not necessary to spend money on specialty foods here at Beauty Boot Camp. I truly believe that eating foods you don't usually eat is the reason that so many diets fail. Don't go too far afield from the foods you and your family enjoy. There are personal and cultural choices in cuisine that cannot be denied.

You can avoid waste by cooking large quantities and then freezing meals in individual or family-sized portions. It's a lot cheaper to make your own sauces and salad dressings, and they'll make your food taste better. You can thin down bottled salad dressings with vinegar and reduce the calories by half. Fruits and vegetables bought while in season are usually cheaper than the packaged variety and they are healthier for you because they are richer in vitamins.

The less expensive cuts of meat are also tastier. They just take a bit more preparation. You should be careful of the more expensive cuts anyway, because they have more fat. If you cook on the grill, buy the least expensive cut you can find. It will still taste great! You can also slash your budget by cutting down on the meat, and doubling up on the vegetables when you are preparing a casserole or stew.

A salad bar is a great take-out choice when you are eating on the run—if you avoid the fatty extras. Go for at least 75 percent greens, and make it dark greens for the most nutrients. Salad bars featuring soups can give you a complete meal for very little money.

You can also reduce the fat in your recipes by making substitutions. Substitute low-fat versions of cheese, milk, sour cream, etc. Sauté vegetables in water or stock instead of oil. You'll be the only one noticing the difference.

Budget Services

If you're looking for an inexpensive haircut, facial, manicure, or pedicure, or even hair coloring, check to see what beauty schools exist in your area. They offer services at very reasonable rates in order to train their students on live models. You're doing them a favor, so they're more than happy to see you.

Don't be nervous about having a student work on you. The trainers are right next to them, guiding them step by step. They will usually take their time with you, and your savings can be as much as 70 percent.

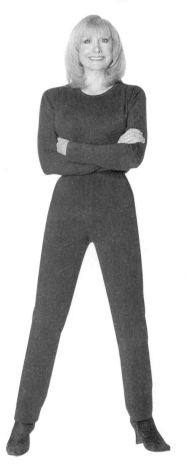

Diane's Tips:

BUDGET WORKOUT

The best workouts are the most economical and the most natural. Walking is free, low-impact, and it's one of the best overall workouts. To prevent boredom, try to choose different routes to vary your scenery.

You'll save money on landscapers and cleaning services when you begin to do your own housework and gardening—and you'll feel a sense of accomplishment. You can create your own mini-gym with inexpensive or common household items, such as a jump rope or an ab "machine" made out of a beach towel. Become your own personal trainer and save the time it would have taken to travel back and forth to a health club.

Put a little steam into every movement you make.

Do lunges while you vacuum.

Use a little extra force when pulling on those pesky weeds.

You'll be getting rid of those jiggly arms and toning the underarm area.

Do squats whenever picking anything up.

Stretch whenever you are reaching into a cabinet.

Use two rags when doing jobs on your hands and knees.

Use vigorous circling motions to work your arms and waist.

Switch to a rotary lawn mower.

Use broad strokes when you are raking the yard.

Get a jump rope. Jumping rope burns fat, defines muscles, and fights cellulite. Plus, it's fun! Try to remember some of those childhood jumping rhymes to get you in the mood.

Fill up soda bottles with water or sand and use them as hand weights.

My Journal:

During the day, keep track of how much you spend, and on what.

My budget today is: _____

List ways you can save money today. Can you pass up the vending machine, bring your lunch to work, or skip a shopping trip?

_____

_____

What purchases do you regularly make that could be trimmed from your budget? Are they rewards to yourself, bad habits, or just things you buy without thinking about it?

_____

_____

_____

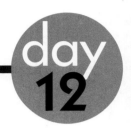

Sometimes measuring the time your regular daily activities take can be a real eye-opener. Today, time the following activities. Comment on what you've learned.

Lunch hour _____

Shower _____

TV viewing time _____

Phone time, business calls _____

Phone time, personal calls _____

Boot Camp Basics:

Travel Basics

There's no reason to let your looks go when you travel. Simplify when you travel, yes. Leave style behind, no.

✓ Pick two wardrobe colors only. This takes a lot of restraint, but it makes packing a matter of minutes, rather than hours.

☐ Keep your suitcase light by paring down on your shoes. You will need one pair of dress heels plus a walking shoe. That's it, unless you're going to a resort where you'll need a pair of sandals.

☐ Use shampoo as a body wash and a detergent for fine washables.

☐ Roll everything you pack for less wrinkling and more space.

❑ Save film containers and use them to pack just the right amount of shampoo, conditioner, jewelry, medication, and other small items.

❑ Pack tightly. Loose clothing quickly wrinkles.

❑ Bring plastic supermarket bags to hold wet and dirty items.

❑ Stuff shoes with belts, hosiery, underwear, and jewelry.

❑ Some items like shampoos and lotions can open under airplane or packing pressure. Pack them in plastic bags.

❑ Button and zipper everything to reduce wrinkling.

day twelve
my diet today

Breakfast: _____
_____

Lunch: _____
_____

Dinner: _____
_____

Snack: _____
_____

Glasses of Water:
☐ ☐ ☐ ☐ ☐ ☐ ☐ ☐ ☐ ☐

Secret Weapons

There's a lot more to top-of-the-line style than just losing weight and changing hairstyles. There are secret weapons in the beauty industry that can give you an extra edge. You can attain that style you've long admired. Have you ever wondered "how did she get that look?" Read on!

Your new look isn't complete unless it comes with a new outlook, discipline, and a lifetime plan. A healthy and happy lifestyle must become an integral part of your plan. The techniques and tools you've been learning will ensure your results will be more permanent and natural.

Become a beauty observer. Appreciate it in the same way you admire flowers or art. When you look at a person, judge the package. That package is made up of details.

Look at a picture of someone who possesses total beauty and style. Now, break the details down. Do this with several pictures, and you'll begin to see similarities in each of the pictures. These details are the ones that you want to finesse. Set a standard for yourself, then stick with it. Visualization is key.

Use visualization to help you establish a style and stick with it. By doing this, you will create a signature style and make maintenance much easier. Create a flow that both looks and feels natural.

Master one technique that will get you noticed and remembered. Create the best eyes or invent a unique way to wear earrings. Strive to honor and learn from other types of beauty. It will generate new ideas, and help you respect your own uniqueness.

Makeup Weapons

The secret weapon of a great face is not only to look good but also to look like you're having a good time. A face has power. Most of us don't realize how much. Women of great style use their faces to express that power. They feel good in their skin and it shows. Everything that goes on your face needs to serve the purpose of revealing that expression.

Foundation evens out your complexion and gives radiance to your skin. You wear just enough to cover flaws, not to mask your face. If you have somehow been among the lucky ones blessed with already beautiful skin, then all you need is a light dusting of powder.

LEARN

THE

SECRET

WEAPONS

OF

THOSE

WHO

MAKE

STYLE

LOOK

EASY.

Concealer works where foundation doesn't. It gets rid of circles under your eyes, broken capillaries, and skin eruptions. Powder sets foundation and gives a smooth finish to your face, eliminating shine. It keeps makeup from wearing off.

Use an eyelash curler to awaken your eyes and give the appearance of a more alert face. It will also make mascara easier to apply. Petroleum jelly allows powdered eye shadow to become cream. It keeps eyebrows groomed, and creates lip gloss out of lipstick, and lipstick out of a lip pencil. Eyeliner brings out eyes and creates definition. Without eyeliner, eyes can look tired and lost. Eyes are best expressed with eyeliner rimmed around the entire eye, and then softened. Mascara gives you the lashes you've dreamed about and frames the eyes. It should be applied from the roots up.

Lip color is a quick way to set the mood for a finished look. Blush gives the face a healthy glow. It also helps shape and "wakes up" the face.

Hair Weapons

Great hair starts with a healthy diet. Shiny, vibrant hair is the result of a diet rich in zinc and vitamin A, which prevents dry hair and scalp. Vitamin B6, found in eggs and other sources, supports protein, which primarily makes up hair.

Protect your hair by conditioning first, then shampooing, then conditioning again. Pretreating your hair is particularly important if your hair is processed or flat-ironed on a frequent basis.

Stay away from flat colors. If you have your hair done professionally, have your stylist give you a combination of highlights and lowlights. They really do look more natural and are flattering to the complexion. If you color at home, consider doing your own highlighting or purchase one of the multi-toned hair colorings that recently have come on the market.

Don't fight with the natural growth of your hair. An experienced stylist should be able to work around cowlicks and curls. Fighting them creates a style that takes too much time and care. You should blow dry your hair in the pattern in which your hair grows. Although blow drying your hair in all directions might dry it faster, the results will be frizzy and untamed.

Use a paddle brush when blow drying, and dry on top of the hair to prevent flyaways. Find a hairbrush with natural bristles (boar bristles are the best). They're kinder to the hair strands and their porosity will absorb oils from your scalp.

Always blow dry on the medium setting. Although it may be tempting to use the highest setting, it can fry your hair. Plus, a medium setting will effectively seal the cuticle, which will keep your hair smooth. A medium heat setting can actually help your hair's condition by allowing conditioners and moisturizers to penetrate into the hair shaft.

Finishing Touch Weapons

The doyennes of style are the women who have an ability to accessorize. I consider finishing an outfit with "just the right piece" a true art. Whether it's a great pair of sunglasses or the perfect handbag, it brings the wearer to the next level. Conversely, the wrong

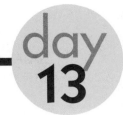

color hose or bad shoes can make an Armani look like a Halloween costume.

There are finishing touch weapons that will extend your wardrobe and bring drab to dazzling.

Always match your shoes and hose when possible. It slims out the legs and looks elegant. Beige shoes with matching beige hose will work with any outfit. Don't date yourself by trying to match your shoes with your outfit.

Choose the best purse you can afford. It's at eye level and makes the quickest impression. Use bracelets to create cuffs and to dress up a watch.

Experiment with pins. They make great necklace enhancers and are lots of fun on a purse. Belts look best when they are the same tone as the outfit.

Take your gold chains and knot them at the neck for an updated look. It will bring flattering light to your face. Be sure to check out flea markets for bargains. Vintage jewelry can really add value to an outfit.

Diet Weapons

Don't be caught without the tricks and tools that will protect you against the daily temptations and challenges you'll face.

For starters, find a belt that fits too snugly to be comfortable. It keeps you aware of why you need to diet and makes you too uncomfortable to overeat. Plus, you will enjoy watching the belt get larger and changing notches. Think of it as natural stomach stapling.

Carry perfume around with you. When you pass a restaurant or bakery where the delightful smells beckon you to come in, hold the perfume to your nose. You could also carry a perfumed hanky. There are very attractive solid perfume compacts that do the job beautifully and inconspicuously.

Drink something warm when your stomach growls. Warm liquids (like teas and boullions) create a feeling of fullness without extra calories.

Dim the lights and slow down the music. Johns Hopkins University has documented a reduction in appetite when dining under low lighting. Bright lights stimulate us psychologically.

Always choose a small plate, the darker the better. It can trick you into believing your plate is fuller than it is. While eating, take deep breaths between bites, and be sure to put your fork down.

Turkey jerky is a high protein, low calorie snack that models keep in their bags for when they need to eat and there's no time to stop. It fills them up, and it takes a long time to chew.

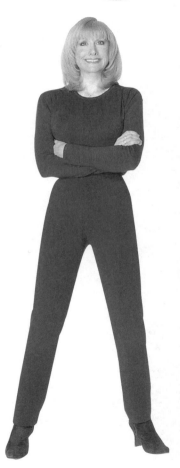

Diane's Tips:

STYLE WEAPONS

—STYLE IS A MUST.—

Pashminas are not style. Capri pants are not style. They're just fashion.

Fashion comes and goes, far too often as far as my budget is concerned.

But there are weapons of style that last long beyond trends.

You can wear each and every fashion trend that comes down the runway and

still never possess a modicum of style. Style means not being afraid to take risks.

STYLE IS HAVING A TRADEMARK

AND BEING ACKNOWLEDGED FOR IT.

These style weapons have been around forever. They're called classics.
You can wear them for the next ten or twenty years. Purchase the highest
quality that you can afford so you won't end up looking for replacements

EVERYONE NEEDS A BASIC BLACK DRESS.

It's the one item you can wear day into night, summer into winter.

Choose your poison: gold hoop earrings or diamond studs.

I know, some decisions are never easy.

Keep a quality black skirt and black trousers in a seasonless wool.

Everyone needs a well-cut jacket. Check the seams and lining to ensure quality.

White cotton shirts never go out of style. Choose men's tailoring.

Don't neglect the classic, clean style of a cotton t-shirt.

Hang onto that cardigan and tank sweater set.

Add the following items to your personal style for versatility.

With the right attitude and proper maintenance, you could live in
these pieces and be totally stylish:

a tank watch • loafers or mules • pearls • a trench coat

My Journal:

Visualize your new look. How do you see these things updating, changing, evolving, and improving after the Beauty Boot Camp is complete?

Face _____

Body _____

Posture _____

Movements _____

List your five most flattering outfits.

1. _____
2. _____
3. _____
4. _____
5. _____

What are your never-fail cosmetics?

1. _____
2. _____
3. _____
4. _____
5. _____

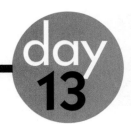

Which of your accessories are the most versatile and foolproof?

1. _____

2. _____

3. _____

4. _____

Create a backup plan for a bad hair day. What alternative styles could you implement in the middle of the day?

1. _____

2. _____

What hair accessories could help the cause?

1. _____

2. _____

What classic pieces of clothing do you need to add to your wardrobe?

1. _____

2. _____

Boot Camp Basics:

Celebrity Basics

Many of your favorite celebrities use great tricks to maintain their terrific looks.

★ When **Daisy Fuentes** needs to drop a few pounds, she drinks one liter of chamomile tea and one liter of water daily. The combination accelerates fat burning.

★ **Cindy Crawford** makes a spritzer out of equal amounts of milk and water. She refreshes her skin with it throughout the day.

★ **Elizabeth Hurley's** secret for staying slim is to eat with smaller utensils. It slows her eating down, which enables reasonable, healthy portions.

★ **Vanna White** stays a svelte 110 pounds at 5'6" by starting her day with oatmeal.

★ Stirring a bit of honey into her tea helps the eternally glamorous **Ann-Margret** stave off her urge for sweets.

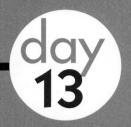

⭐ ***Jennifer Lopez*** concentrates on grains as the mainstay of her diet.

⭐ ***Julia Roberts*** sometimes uses personal trainers, but her favorite way to exercise is privately with her collection of exercise videos.

⭐ Soap opera actress ***Susan Lucci's*** favorite snack is sardines. She eats them for their omega-3 fatty acids, which are essential for smooth skin.

⭐ ***Jane Seymour*** enjoys diet popsicles for her sweet treats.

⭐ ***Sarah Jessica Parker*** uses rose hip oil under her eyes to combat wrinkling.

⭐ Model/actress ***Tyra Banks*** jogs three miles a day to combat flab.

day thirteen
my diet today

Breakfast: _____
_____

Lunch: _____
_____

Dinner: _____
_____

Snack: _____
_____

Glasses of Water:
☐ ☐ ☐ ☐ ☐ ☐ ☐ ☐ ☐ ☐

Maintenance Maneuvers

KEEP

ON

THE

PATH

TO

THE

NEW,

BEAUTIFUL

YOU.

Now that you've reached the last day of Beauty Boot Camp, it's time to figure out how to maintain all that you've learned and accomplished. It's my hope that the time you've spent on this program has been one of self-discovery and improvement. I hope that along with the beauty tips you've learned, you've also learned to honor yourself.

You need to ask yourself now if you feel any different. Hopefully you are feeling more in control of your life, your body, and your surroundings. You should also feel more in tune with your body. You should have learned tangible skills that you're using on a daily basis. Take a moment to note these feelings and skills in your journal. You'll want to capture this personal information and refer to it in the future if you feel the urge to go off track.

You should now possess both the courage and the skills to change your body, mind, and spirit when you're not getting the results you desire. You should also have a relationship of respect with your body so that it, in return, will function exquisitely for you.

Now that you know how to eat, how to treat your body, and how to nurture your psyche, you will feel obligated to do so.

If you've made a dramatic transformation, then you've pushed yourself further than you ever before pushed yourself. Beauty, exercise, and diet take work and time. No one is born beautiful and no one stays beautiful without committing that time and attention. Models and celebrities have used the Beauty Boot Camp program time and time again because it works for them. You can also use it as a safety net to fall back on when life throws you a curve.

Home Maintenance

I don't care how old you are, keep things around that remind you of the best times of your life. The more pleasant your surroundings, the less stress will seep into them. By keeping souvenirs of your life, you will never be lonely. You are at home with yourself.

Don't worry about maintaining the perfect home or feel like you have failed if you are unable to replicate the pages of *House Beautiful*. The late *Vogue* editor Diana Vreeland once said, "A little bad taste is like a splash of paprika. It's hearty, it's healthy, it's physical."

Let your surroundings reflect your joy of living and your fun-loving spirit. Start collections and display them prominently. Don't save your treasures for special occasions. Every day should be treated as a special day.

Add color into your home where you can. Red energizes, orange promotes joy and brings confidence, yellow lifts the spirit, green provides balance, and blue promotes relaxation and peace.

Grow herbs in your kitchen. You'll enjoy their fresh, chemical-free tastes. Many stores sell inexpensive herb kits that you simply open up and water.

Body Maintenance

You can maintain your diet and exercise regime with more ease if it fits into your lifestyle. Keep a record book in your bathroom and write down your weight and body measurements on a monthly basis to stay on track.

Do everything you can to maintain at least thirty minutes of exercise a day. If you work long hours, try to take a walk at lunch and eat at your desk. Walking will also prevent leg cramping. Get up and stretch, push against the back of your chair to work your arms. Back up against a wall and improve your posture and your buttocks with a few squats.

Center your diet around each of the four main food groups, and try to include five portions of vegetables and fruits every day. Continuing to drink eight to ten glasses of ice water a day will help keep you full and maintain your weight. Don't stop just because Boot Camp is over.

Also, remember to schedule your beauty sleep so that you're getting nine hours a night. Before heading to bed, make a list of the next day's activities. Knowing that you're organized will allow you to rest a little more easily.

Do some deep breathing exercises while you're in bed to induce sleep. Lie flat and breathe slowly and deeply in and out of your nostrils. Starting with your feet, tighten and release each muscle in your body. Feel your body growing heavier and heavier, sinking deeper into the mattress.

Beauty Maintenance

Take beauty with you wherever you go and consider it an integral part of being properly dressed and well groomed. Your beauty maintenance should be as natural to you as brushing your teeth. Beyond allowing you to look good, it should make you feel good about yourself.

You'll have good beauty days and bad beauty days. Rather than obsessing over what's wrong, focus on what's working. You'll draw strength from your beauty knowledge and learn to combat problems as they come up. You'll follow the blueprint that you've mastered in Beauty Boot Camp and improvise and adapt it by using your own creativity.

Stay true to your own beauty system. Be aware of what works for you and throw away what doesn't. When you don't feel your beauty inside, external success is impossible.

You're now aware that there are no beauty miracles. It takes time and patience. The results will be worth the investment of both. It also takes some practice. Learning how to be more beautiful should be both fun and self-gratifying.

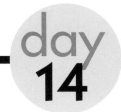

Occasionally, you should take a day of rest from beauty maintenance. I'm not suggesting that you neglect to comb your hair or leave traces of makeup on from the night before. But from time to time, do only the minimum. Cleanse and moisturize your face, pull your hair back, and try not to feel guilty about it. Such a day will likely cause you to miss the beauty and style you've incorporated into your life. You'll miss the pleasure of looking in the mirror and fully appreciating your look and your knowledge.

Excellence comes with time. It's never too early to start, and never too late to learn. There's no amount of cosmetics that can work on a woman who doesn't like herself. Your face is a canvas, but you can't paint on someone else's face.

Style Maintenance

Here's the number one rule in style maintenance: unless you love it, don't wear it, use it, or own it. Once you've discovered your individual style, you have the freedom to be yourself. Fashion fads won't pass you by. You'll simply choose to ignore them.

Of course, fashion is fun and you'll want to occasionally give in to the whimsy of it. But you'll always return to the tried and true, to what looks and works best for your body type and personality. You'll still be perceived as an up-to-date and stylish woman.

You will take the best of today and mix it with the successes of yesterday. Finding and maintaining your style will not only save you a great deal of money and time, but it will provide you with a sense of security. You'll stand out in the most positive way. You'll be expressing your imagination and individuality.

Life Maintenance

Where would you like to be in the next month, in the next year, and in the next ten years?

It is my hope that you have been able to make a dream, or at least part of your dream, come true, and that you'll continue to dream and create. If this has been a jumpstart for you, I hope that you will come back to Beauty Boot Camp for reinforcement, as well as the occasional tune-up. It's a busy world out there, and it's easy to lose touch with your inner self when the outer world is beckoning and burgeoning.

Try something new every day: a new food, a new color, a new way to connect with your body and mind. Your relationship with the world will only be worth the quality of the relationship you have with yourself. You must be as patient and forgiving of yourself as you hopefully are with others.

Share your knowledge with others. Don't let the beauty bashers get to you. Gather up your friends and have a beauty day, or a pajama party home spa. There is no age, weight, or stereotype to beauty. Give to others and let them give back to you. Do the best you can and enjoy your life.

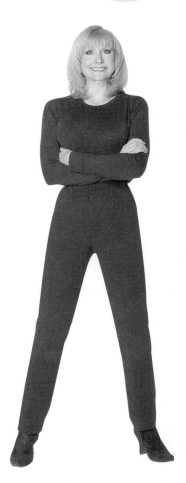

Diane's Tips:

HAIR REMOVAL MANEUVERS

Although **shaving** is never fun, taking a little extra time will make it easier, as well as result in a smoother look and feel.

For starters, always thoroughly moisten hair before shaving. Hair conditioner works much better than shaving cream. It gets the hair standing up so that it is easier to reach. To make a shave last longer, use a **loofah** or a coarse washcloth just before. This helps to shed the top layer of dead skin, and removes oil and perspiration for a much closer shave.

Use a fresh twin blade razor to reduce drag on your skin and prevent red, blotchy, and irritated skin. You may want to consider a razor with a replaceable blade. They have heavier handles, usually allowing for a closer shave with a lighter touch.

Leave **hard-to-shave** spots for last. This gives the more difficult areas, such as the knees and the back of the thighs a chance to soften.

Shave in the opposite direction from the hair growth. It prevents hair from curling under the skin and becoming ingrown.

The **bikini area** is, without a doubt, the most difficult to shave because the hair grows in various directions. There are some women who prefer to use a beard trimmer in this area. It leaves no unsightly red bumps, and it is safe when used at its lowest setting.

If **waxing** is your hair removal technique of choice, don't shave or use a depilatory at least two weeks before waxing. It's also important not to wax around the time of your menstrual period when your skin is more puffy. It helps to exfoliate between waxings to slough off dead skin that can clog pores.

After shaving or waxing, treat **ingrown hairs** with alcohol to avoid infection and red bumps. Any raw looking areas can be treated with tea tree oil.

My Journal:

In what ways are you different from anyone else?

_____

_____

In our fourteen days together, what did you achieve?

_____

_____

What do you need to continue to work on?

_____

_____

What was easiest?

_____

What was most difficult and why?

_____

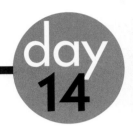

Weighing In

Weight

_____

Waist

_____

Hips

_____

Bust

_____

Thighs

_____

Where do you see yourself in a month?

_____

_____

In a year?

_____

_____

Five years?

_____

_____

Today, you may wish to take a picture of yourself and paste it in your journal. In a month, a year, or five years, come back and see how fabulous you looked and felt at the end of Boot Camp. If you want to come back and see me again, begin at Day One. A refresher course never hurts!

Model Basics

A model's bag is filled with basics that take them through the day looking and feeling picture perfect.

☑ Baby wipes are a great tool for both cleansing the face and removing makeup. Baby wipes are hygienic and gentle on the face. Most versions contain lanolin, which is a skin softener. They can also remove stains and deodorant streaks.

☐ Hemorrhoid cream can be used to reduce the swelling of puffy eyes, double chins, and puffy cheeks. It can be used to temporarily smooth out cellulite.

☐ Use white eyeliner along the lash line and under the brow to create a wide-eyed look.

☐ Ripped pantyhose can be recycled into hair scrunchies. Cut them into three- or four-inch widths and hold hair back without stress or split ends. Opaque hose has more elasticity.

❏ Hair spray misted lightly on pantyhose makes them more run resistant. Also, spray it on a finger and pat gently on your eyebrows to keep them in place.

❏ Teething rings placed on the eyes will take away puffiness and give them a more alert appearance. Place them in a glass of ice water for five minutes before using.

❏ Shea butter can be used on dry skin to prevent stretch marks.

❏ Fabric softener sheets get rid of static cling and smooth out hair frizzies.

❏ Metal spoons run under cold water soothe tired eyes and reduce swelling in puffy areas.

day fourteen
my diet today

Breakfast: _____
_____

Lunch: _____
_____

Dinner: _____
_____

Snack: _____
_____

Glasses of Water:
☐ ☐ ☐ ☐ ☐ ☐ ☐ ☐ ☐ ☐

Before I Leave You

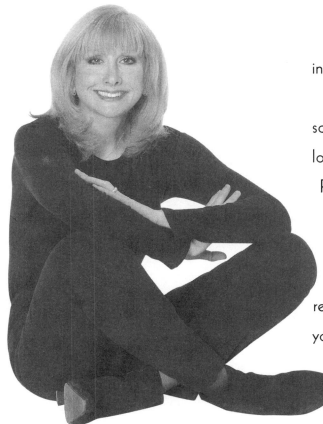

It has been such an honor to be your leader in this Beauty Boot Camp program.

I hope that you have been able to make some important changes to your weight, your looks, and most importantly, your life. Remember, Beauty Boot Camp is here whenever you need to bring yourself to the next level of your being.

Your fitness and beauty should be realistic and enjoyable. It should contribute to your well-being, not overwhelm it. Do the very best you can with all of your gifts.

Then use them to add to the many adventures awaiting you in life.

About the Author

Bestselling author **Diane Irons** is America's favorite beauty expert. A model since the age of thirteen and an internationally-acclaimed image expert, she has transformed models and celebrities throughout the world.

She has appeared on national radio and TV including *The View*, *Good Morning America*, *Sally Jesse Raphael*, QVC, CNN, CNBC, *CBS This Morning*, *Entertainment Tonight*, *Inside Edition*, *Fox News*, *Maury Povich*, *Montel Williams*, Lifetime, and Discovery.

She has been featured in *Cosmopolitan*, *Allure*, the *Wall Street Journal*, the *New York Post*, the *Chicago Tribune*, and the *Los Angeles Times*. She is a regular contributor to *Woman's World* and eDiets.com.

Visit Diane's website
at www.dianeirons.com
or email her at dianeirons@aol.com

You can write to her in care of:
Sourcebooks, Inc.
P.O. Box 4410
Naperville, IL 60567

Index